FRHS

Management Mistakes in Healthcare

This book defines management mistakes and offers a variety of models to classify and interpret them. It describes the evolution of management mistakes, techniques for identifying and disclosing mistakes, the relationship between management and medical mistakes, and steps to prevent and correct them. Seven case studies, drawn from a real set of events in healthcare organizations, describe management mistakes and are followed by commentaries by experts in the field of healthcare management, indicating measures that might have produced more positive outcomes.

Ultimately, managers will not be completely successful in making healthcare better and more cost-effective without viewing mistakes as learning opportunities. This book is written for healthcare managers throughout the world and for the benefit of their patients, staff, and communities.

Paul B. Hofmann, P. H., FACHE, Provenance Health Partners, Moraga, California, provides consulting services to healthcare systems and hospitals. He has served as Executive Vice President and COO of the Alta Bates Corporation, a non-profit healthcare system in northern California, Executive Director of Emory University Hospital in Atlanta, Georgia, and Director of Stanford University Hospital and Clinics. In addition to being co-editor of *Managing Ethically: An Executive Guide* (Health Administration Press, 2001), he is the author of over 125 articles and has held faculty appointments at Harvard, UCLA, Stanford, Emory, and the University of California.

Frankie Perry, R. N., M. A., FACHE®, currently serves on the faculty of the University of New Mexico and as the Executive Director of The Chairman's Society, an Atlanta-based organization whose mission is the education and training of healthcare board Chairmen-Officers. She has served as Assistant Medical Center Director of Hurley Medical Center in Flint, Michigan. In addition to her hospital experience, she served as Executive Vice President of the American College of Healthcare Executives and as a national and international healthcare management consultant with engagements in Cairo, Egypt, Doha, Qatar, and Bombay, India, among others. She is the author of *The Tracks We Leave. Ethics in Healthcare Management*, published in 2001.

Management Mistakes in Healthcare

Identification, Correction, and Prevention

Edited by

Paul B. Hofmann and Frankie Perry

Foreword by

Richard J. Davidson

President, American Hospital Association

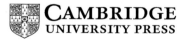

CAMBRIDGE
UNIVERSITY PRESS

PUBLISHED BY THE PRESS SYNDICATE OF THE UNIVERSITY OF CAMBRIDGE
The Pitt Building, Trumpington Street, Cambridge, United Kingdom

CAMBRIDGE UNIVERSITY PRESS
The Edinburgh Building, Cambridge, CB2 2RU, UK
40 West 20th Street, New York, NY 10011–4211, USA
477 Williamstown Road, Port Melbourne, VIC 3207, Australia
Ruiz de Alarcón 13, 28014 Madrid, Spain
Dock House, The Waterfront, Cape Town 8001, South Africa

http://www.cambridge.org

First published 2005

Printed in the United Kingdom at the University Press, Cambridge

Typeface in Minion 10.5/14pt system Advent 3b2 8.01 [TB]

A catalog record for this book is available from the British Library

Library of Congress Cataloging in Publication data

Hofmann, Paul B., 1941 –
Mistakes in healthcare management : indentification, correction, and prevention/Paul
Hofmann & Frankie Perry.
  p. cm.
Includes bibliographical references and index.
ISBN 0-521-82900-3
1. Health services administration.   2. Health services administration–Case studies.
I. Perry, Frankie.   II. Title.
RA971.H56   2004
362.1'068–dc22   2004051861

ISBN 0 521 82900 3   hardback

Contents

Notes on the contributors

Paul B. Hofmann, Dr. P. H., FACHE, Provenance Health Partners, Moraga, California, has over 35 years of experience in healthcare consulting, hospital administration and teaching. Prior to providing performance improvement consulting services to health systems and hospitals, he served as Executive Vice President and COO of the Alta Bates Corporation, a non-profit healthcare system in northern California; Executive Director of Emory University Hospital in Atlanta, Georgia; and Director of Stanford University Hospital and Clinics in Palo Alto, California. In addition to being co-editor of *Managing Ethically: An Executive's Guide* (Health Administration Press, 2001) he is the management ethics consultant to the American College of Healthcare Executives and author of over 125 publications. Dr. Hofmann has held faculty appointments at Harvard, UCLA, Stanford, Emory, the University of California, and Seton Hall University.

Frankie Perry, R. N., FACHE®, has held senior-level positions in both nursing and hospital administration and brings many years of healthcare management experience to her co-authorship of this volume. In addition to her hospital experience, she served as Executive Vice President of the American College of Healthcare Executives and as a national and international healthcare management consultant. She is a widely published author of articles on ethics and healthcare management and was a 1984 recipient of the Edgar C. Hayhow Award for Article of the Year by the American College of Hospital Administrators. Her most recent book is *The Tracks We Leave: Ethics in Healthcare Management*, (Health Administration Press, 2001). She currently serves on the faculty of the University of New Mexico and as the Executive Director of The Chairman's Society, an Atlanta-based organization whose mission is the education and training of healthcare board Chairmen-Officers.

Carol Bayley is Vice President for Ethics and Justice Education at Catholic Healthcare West in San Francisco. She has published in the areas of alternative medicine, the philosophy of science, pharmacy ethics, genetics, and medical error and is an Adjunct Faculty Member at the University of San Francisco.

Robert S. Bonney, J. D., FACHE, is Senior Vice President for Business Development for the Saint Luke's Health System in Kansas City, Missouri. He is a prolific author and holds faculty positions at the University of Missouri and the University of Kansas.

Fred L. Brown, FACHE, was founder, President, and CEO of BJC Healthcare in Saint Louis, Missouri and currently serves as Chairman of the National Kidney Foundation and as Vice Chairman of the Board of Commissioners of the Joint Commission on Accreditation of Healthcare Organizations.

Emily Friedman, an internationally recognized writer, lecturer, and health policy and ethics analyst based in Chicago, is also Adjunct Assistant Professor at the Boston University School of Public Health.

Joyce A. Godwin had twenty-five years experience in healthcare management before she decided to pursue corporate governance interests. She now lives in Albuquerque, New Mexico and serves on numerous local, national, and international corporate and healthcare boards.

Benn Greenspan, MPH, Ph.D., FACHE, recently retired after serving as President and CEO of Sinai Health System of Chicago for thirteen years. He consults and serves as clinical associate professor and director of the MHA Program at the University of Illinois, School of Public Health.

Wanda J. Jones, MPH, is President of New Century Healthcare Institute, a non-profit organization devoted to research, development, and education in healthcare delivery, located in San Francisco.

Trudy Land, FACHE, is a consultant providing executive healthcare services. She has more than twenty years of experience in healthcare administration and management. Ms. Land is the recipient of several healthcare honors and awards.

Mark R. Neaman, FACHE, is the President and CEO of Evanston Northwestern Healthcare Corporation, Evanston, Illinois. He is also a past chairman of the Board of Governors of the American College of Healthcare Executives.

Robert Nicholls, a former senior NHS executive, is now Chairman of the National Clinical Assessment Authority in the United Kingdom and a lay member of the General Medical Council.

Ruth M. Rothstein recently retired as Chief of the Cook County Bureau of Health Services, Chicago, Illinois, and has led the Bureau since its creation in 1991. She is widely known and highly regarded throughout the country for her leadership and creativity in improving the quality of the healthcare system.

John A. Russell, MHA, FACHE, served as the CEO for the Hospital Association of Pennsylvania for some twenty-two years and previously held senior administrative positions at academic medical centers associated with Northwestern University, University of Wisconsin, and Pennsylvania State University.

Andrew Wall, B. A, M.Sc, FIHM, a former NHS Chief Executive, is now a part-time lecturer at the Health Services Management Centre, University of Birmingham, United Kingdom. His numerous publications include *Ethics and the Health Services Manager* and *The Reorganized National Health Service*.

John Abbott Worthley, D. P. A., based in Glen Cove, New York, is an international consultant and Professor of Public Management in the United States and Asia. He is the author of *Organizational Ethics in the Compliance Context, The Ethics of the Ordinary in Healthcare,* and several other books.

Foreword

Dick Davidson

President, American Hospital Association

Reading for the first time the hard-hitting case studies in this important book took me back to my days as a young school teacher in Delaware. On Monday nights, I'd watch the hospital drama "Ben Casey." As the show opened, a wise old voice would intone "man, woman, birth, death, infinity." On screen, an anonymous right hand holding a stubby piece of chalk drew the universal symbol for each word on a classroom blackboard. Shot in black and white, the show was gritty and real, and it made Ben Casey's County General Hospital seem like a metaphor for the world the rest of us lived in.

In fact, hospitals once were perceived as a much more integral part of the community than they are today. And this image has been reinforced for decades by our popular culture. In the 1970s, we had kindly Marcus Welby, MD, treating patients at, appropriately, Hope Memorial. In the 1980s, hard-luck patients were warmly welcomed at city-owned St. Elsewhere.

These dramas showed hometown American hospitals as the public saw them – life-saving, compassionate and participating partners in their community. Week after week, the familiar characters showed us how the life and death consequences of healthcare bind us in a very special relationship to the people and institutions that care for us. The shows were huge hits because they validated the real-world experiences of ordinary people when they went to the hospital.

But, as we neared the twenty-first century, forces shaping how the public sees hospitals were changing. Public opinion research showed that more and more Americans felt that our healthcare system wasn't meeting their needs. A stream of negative news reports played up worst-case medical errors, billing inequities, and the immense problems of a system becoming more expensive and complex. On TV, the doctors and nurses on "ER" still seemed heroic, but the hospital seemed like a bureaucratic barrier that got in the way of good people trying to help people.

What had changed? Was art really imitating life? Research told us that the public was experiencing a widening healthcare *confidence chasm*. The public worried about quality, safety, and their ability to afford the care they might need if they lost precious health insurance. The public clearly wanted a more personal, less business-focused healthcare system.

Not surprisingly, out of the spotlight, policy makers, lawmakers and the dedicated men and women who run our hospitals and health systems have wrestled with these same issues. But their successful efforts to address these concerns have received little attention. After all, why kill a good story line? There is little tension or drama in the often slow and careful path of change.

The uncovered good news is that successful change is radically reducing clinical errors and producing better clinical outcomes. The words "patient safety" are more than a mere term of clinical art; they are rallying cry for the nationwide movement to transform healthcare itself. Hospitals have committed enormous human and financial resources to the cause.

But overlooked and understudied – until this book – is a lesser-known and seldom examined area in which quality improvement can make all the difference – the kind of *executive* errors and *management* mistakes that can also devastate a hospital's performance, reputation, and public standing. Also overlooked and understudied – until this book – is what we can do to correct and prevent them. And the bottom line? This, too, needs to be a cause.

"Executive error" often occurs out of the media's line of sight. It's easy to pass by, especially when the public spotlight shines so brightly on our national effort to reduce medical errors. Unfortunately, some organizational cultures prefer it that way, shortsightedly choosing plausible deniability to honest and transparent accountability. And similar to clinical error, the world of management error is often characterized by a dysfunctional culture of blame, shame, and punishment.

Now, thanks to editors Paul Hofmann and Frankie Perry and an outstanding assembly of contributing authors, a sharply focused and bright new spotlight is illuminating this long-ignored subject. Hofmann and Perry, experts on healthcare management practices and ethics, teach us here about the up-close forces and factors that trigger executive errors in the first place. They set up the challenges that confront healthcare leaders who need to understand the landscape as it appears from 30,000 feet. The lessons to be learned from the seven cases they present are urgent and vital for all hospital and health systems executives and their management teams, employees, and patients.

As you'll see in the pages that follow, this is a tough area to investigate. In an atmosphere of blame and shame, the old rules impose zero tolerance for errors and zero tolerance for the humans who err. When a mistake occurs, the shame system contracts in self-defense, and there are scapegoats and punishment, typically with demotion or dismissal. The system, thus "fixed," resumes business as usual. But it remains blind to its inherent failings and in denial over its fatal flaws – until someone errs again.

Internally, the damage can be lethal and lasting. The culture can turn mean and threatening. Teamwork, critical to preventing or fixing management error, crumbles under the weight of self-protection.

Externally, the chain of public trust, tremendously difficult to forge over time, is ever more stressed. The most successful hospital executives and managers take this on faith. Clinical errors? Correct them, learn from them, and move on. Management mistakes? Same thing. Correct them, learn from them, and move on, as well.

Many hospitals are already models for how to succeed in a post-blame and shame era. They know that you don't need to go to business school to apply some common sense. We tell our kids that we learn from our mistakes. We need to practice the same principle in healthcare management. Other important principles you'll take away from this book include:

- Realizing mistakes are not a "people" problem, but a "systems" problem.
- Benefiting from the experience of the patient safety movement.
- Emulating the best practices of hospitals that are "winners."
- Instilling a new culture of teamwork, self-examination and public accountability.
- Improving the quality and diversity of the workforce.
- Capitalizing on the changing demographics of management ranks.
- Balancing an internal business model with a commitment to the community.
- Maintaining good relations with various publics.
- Sharing important information with the community.
- Understanding that hospitals are agents for social change in their communities.

If we follow these principles, we will identify, correct, and prevent management mistakes with the same relentless honesty, vigor, and staying power that we already bring to reducing medical errors.

In the chapters that follow, you'll be reminded that the trust of the public is a precious asset; it accumulates slowly as the public realizes it is safe to invest its faith and good will. Securing and retaining the trust of the public is as high a priority as any hospital can set. Lose this trust through avoidable mistakes and miscalculations, and the price to be paid is more than our system can bear. For this reason alone, even if a hospital's connection to the community already is strong, it must be bolstered. If it is weak, it must be strengthened. If it is broken, it must be fixed.

The world of healthcare is much more complex and intimidating than in the old days of TV's Hope Memorial and St. Elsewhere. The leaders, executives, and management teams running America's healthcare organizations need to remind themselves, their communities, and the entire nation of the true character of America's hospitals, of what we believe, and how we live those beliefs. This is the real value of this book. If we are, indeed, who we say we are, the public's trust fully will be ours. It had better be – Ben Casey's grandkids are counting on it.

Dick Davidson
Washington, DC
August 2004

Preface

Acknowledging and examining mistakes in healthcare management is not a pleasant or popular activity. Although clinical errors have received increasing attention, executive errors have been largely ignored.

Our book is intended as a first step to address this lamentable gap in both the healthcare literature and professional consciousness. By recognizing and reducing clinical errors, healthcare organizations have improved not only the quality of care but also clinical outcomes. Additional benefits can be achieved from similar scrutiny on the administrative side if we are candid about management mistakes and become much more diligent in correcting and preventing them. Through a combination of chapters and cases, along with commentaries, we want to stimulate current managers in hospitals and other healthcare organizations to learn from their previous mistakes and to become more systematic in avoiding their recurrence.

We begin by admitting that a management mistake is not always easy to recognize and define, and that some mistakes are unavoidable. The sources and causes of errors are, however, very clear. Furthermore, as in medicine, mistakes can be the result of acts of omission as well as commission. Disclosing mistakes and developing effective coping techniques are emphasized as essential prerequisites to improving management performance.

John Abbott Worthley (chapter 2) explores the context of management mistakes by distinguishing eight major aspects: legal, organizational, financial, political, professional, ethical, social, and psychological. He provides a robust conceptual framework for understanding and addressing mistakes.

In chapter 3, Wanda J. Jones focuses on a number of critical factors involved in identifying and classifying mistakes, dissecting and divulging them, and dealing with the fear of retribution. Throughout her discussion, she provides vivid examples of management mistakes and their consequences.

Because medical and executive errors usually occur within a complex organizational setting, Carol Bayley (chapter 4) suggests that management can benefit by drawing on the insights produced by the longer history and more extensive experience of clinicians in dealing with their mistakes. Contrasting the "blame and shame" approach with a newer understanding of responsibility for error reduction, she explains why and how cultural issues can play such a critical role.

John A. Russell and Benn Greenspan (chapter 5) draw on their respective backgrounds in managing large and diverse healthcare organizations to provide the reader with an effective framework to deal with the inevitability of executive errors. Their approach is based on lessons learned from personal and career examples of management mistakes, and they offer recommendations designed to correct and avoid mistakes, and to reduce their impact.

Ultimately, according to Emily Friedman (chapter 6), confronting management mistakes is a matter of accepting accountability. She explores the psychology of accountability, discusses the implications of various scandals in both the healthcare and non-healthcare industries, and proposes specific steps for producing accountable leaders and establishing accountable organizations.

These six chapters provide a comprehensive overview of the problems created by management mistakes in healthcare and how they can be identified, corrected, and prevented. Each chapter includes brief descriptions of various mistakes, small and large.

Circumstances associated with a particular situation are almost always complicated by a host of political and other considerations, and the mistakes are rarely the result of only one decision. Consequently, to illustrate these complexities, seven cases (prepared by Frankie Perry and based upon actual events but in fictitious institutions) are presented, followed by commentaries from leaders in the field (chapters 7–13). These leaders were asked to answer the following questions: (1) What management mistakes occurred in this case? (2) How could they have been avoided? (3) What steps could be taken within this organization to prevent these kinds of mistakes in the future? To determine whether the cases and their analyses were relevant to healthcare executives in the United Kingdom, we also asked two distinguished UK experts to provide their perspective (chapter 14).

In our concluding chapter 15, we highlight common themes, offer some admonitions, and suggest why and how examining management mistakes can make a significant difference in the delivery of healthcare. Given the absence of research and the paucity of publications concerning this important issue, we hope others will be motivated to pursue the topic further.

Acknowledgments

We are grateful for this opportunity to address a topic that has not received the attention it deserves. In addition to thanking our colleagues who generously agreed to serve as contributing authors, we want to convey our sincere appreciation for the time and candor of others who were willing to describe management mistakes that formed the basis of our case studies. We are also thankful for the invaluable assistance of Pauline Graham, Commissioning Editor, Science, Technology and Medicine, and Barbara Docherty, our copy-editor, at Cambridge University Press.

Part I

Addressing management mistakes in healthcare

Acknowledging and examining management mistakes

Paul B. Hofmann

Provenance Health Partners, Moraga, California

The failed merger of the hospitals owned by Stanford University and the University of California at San Francisco cost both institutions a combined financial loss of $176 million over a twenty-nine-month period (Russell 2000), but the non-financial costs remain immeasurable. Like all aborted mergers, it was originally well intentioned. However, unlike most mistakes, the failure was highly scrutinized and publicized.

Although the examination of medical errors in the USA was greatly accelerated by the Institute of Medicine (1999) report, *To Err Is Human: Building a Safer Health System*, and physicians have urged colleagues to acknowledge mistakes for years (Hilfiker 1984), the healthcare literature has rarely addressed or even acknowledged *executive* mistakes.

Unsuccessful consolidations, as well as the apparent inability of other mergers to achieve cost-saving targets (Costello 2000), have contributed to a continuing perception that healthcare resources should be better managed. In part, such problems have caused a deterioration of public trust in hospitals, but this erosion has been under way for some time (Hofmann 1991). Ultimately, a reduction in management mistakes should lead to greater public trust, stronger executive performance, improved financial results, enhanced quality of patient care, and higher staff morale. It is difficult to imagine a more compelling set of incentives for aggressively pursuing an analysis and reduction in management mistakes.

In an exceptional article entitled "Morally Managing Medical Mistakes," Smith and Forster (2000) noted that medical mistakes might be simple and benign, cause serious but reversible harm, or result in permanent damage or death. The authors raised a cluster of questions, including: What counts as a mistake or an error? What are the reasons for, and causes of, mistakes? What happens to professionals,

An earlier version of this chapter was previously published in *Frontiers of Health Services Management* 18(2), Spring 2002.

Management Mistakes in Healthcare, ed. Paul Hofmann and Frankie Perry. Published by Cambridge University Press. © Cambridge University Press 2005.

emotionally and spiritually, when mistakes are made? Should mistakes be routinely disclosed, and to whom? All of these inquiries are clearly relevant, but they cover only part of the healthcare landscape. Healthcare administrators also make errors; some are strategic, some may be unethical, and some are inevitable when managing large and very complex service enterprises. As in medicine, the moral imperative is to learn from our mistakes so we can lessen the probability of repeating them. For institutions striving to be learning organizations (Garvin 2000), mistakes could also be viewed as opportunities for promoting individual growth and development.

An understandable reticence

For many reasons, healthcare executives have been reluctant to talk or write about their failures and what they learned from them. Depending on the consequences resulting from a mistake, executives may fear reprimand, job loss, or even legal exposure. In addition, given human nature, pride, and ego, it is understandable that executives have not felt motivated to describe their misjudgments, tactical errors, or blunders. To preserve their sense of self-worth or the illusion of management omniscience, they may contend that uncontrollable events conspired to cause the failure, declaring, "If not for pressures created by limited resources, conflicting opinions, severe time constraints, and uncertain market conditions, I would have made a different and better decision."

However, it is precisely when challenging circumstances raise the stakes of a critical management decision that executives should demonstrate their administrative competence and courage. Most managers can "look good" when the environment is relatively stable and benign. Greenspan (2002) properly notes that the conundrum most frequently confronted by executives is not a decision involving a right and wrong choice, but one pertaining to unappealing options or two attractive alternatives, each with competing sets of values. Nonetheless, displaying organizational aptitude and skill in making the tough calls correctly is one of the major reasons most senior executives are well compensated.

Understandably, mistakes cannot be managed unless they are recognized. Eventually, most errors such as the following, become evident:
- an incompetent manager was tolerated for an inordinate length of time
- negative financial results were not promptly disclosed
- a merger was ill-advised, poorly planned, and/or badly implemented
- managed care contracts were signed without adequate due diligence
- substandard clinical performance by a physician, nurse, or other clinician was not quickly addressed.

Alternatively, there could be doubt or disagreement that an error had occurred. An objective third party could legitimately conclude that a bad outcome was unfortunate, but not necessarily the result of a mistake given the prevailing circumstances. Examples abound: the purchase of physician practices seemed reasonable at the time, as did the decision to acquire that managed care plan, buy the new computer system, sign all those managed care contracts, and hire that candidate for Vice President of Professional Services who interviewed so well and whose credentials and references were impressive.

Defining and acknowledging executive mistakes

Clearly defining an executive error is not easy. What constitutes a mistake, and from whose perspective? In some cases, it may be ambiguous, such as authorizing an interest-free housing loan to help recruit a new chief operating officer. In other instances, it may be clear, such as a CEO obtaining a check for a down payment on his own home from the chief financial officer without board approval. How does one differentiate between the use of poor judgment and sound decision-making processes that simply result in decisions that "don't work out"? Some mistakes are minor or questionable, and others are major and indisputable. Mistakes might thus be viewed on a continuum with shades of gray. Because management is a less precise science than medicine – where, for example, ordering the wrong medication or failing to initiate treatment despite repeated abnormal laboratory findings is an unequivocal error – the management continuum is longer and less exact.

The words "mistake" and "error" have so many connotations that a framework is needed to clarify one's use of the terms. The 1999 Institute of Medicine report defined an error "as the failure of a planned action to be completed as intended or the use of a wrong plan to achieve an end." For purposes of this discussion, a mistake is viewed as *making a decision to act or not act without thoroughly assessing known evidence and incorporating stakeholders' perspectives when the action or inaction (a) places patients, staff, the organization, and/or the community at risk, or (b) is costly to implement, or (c) costly to change.* Often, but not always, such mistakes result in obviously bad outcomes. At least three categories can be identified using this conceptualization: negligence, decisions or non-decisions producing bad outcomes that were neither intended nor foreseeable, and mistakes that do not produce bad outcomes:

• *Negligence* must satisfy several requirements. First, the decision made or action taken is one that a reasonable person would consider risky. Second, a bad outcome occurs. Third, the risky behavior is the proximate cause of the bad outcome. Fourth, a reasonable person would have foreseen such an outcome. Unless all these conditions are present, negligence has not occurred. Negligence is evident when an executive decides not to check the references of a candidate for vice president who has falsified her employment history and, after hiring the person, finds that the individual has embezzled funds for the third time.

- The category of *unintended and unforeseeable bad outcomes* is more self-explanatory. Sometimes, and only in retrospect, perhaps after days, months, or years, a decision or non-decision may be described as a "mistake," and the more substantial the fallout, the greater the interest in holding someone accountable. If best management practices were followed prior to a failed merger or a belated decision to merge, this would be an example of a mistake that was not the result of negligence nor quickly obvious.

- Some might claim that when a mistake does not result in a bad outcome, no error has actually occurred. However, mistakes that do not produce bad outcomes should not be seen as irrelevant or inconsequential, but actually "near misses" or *intercepted mistakes* that can provide invaluable learning experiences. For example, a contingency plan should have been prepared to address a possible shortfall in reimbursement, but legislative intervention and an improvement in payer mix made significant cost reduction measures unnecessary.

Intentional wrongdoing is purposely excluded from this overview. Whether motivated by anger, intimidation, greed, indifference, or other impulses, there is no confusion or ambiguity in such situations; the decision or behavior is unequivocally unacceptable and inappropriate. Such decisions or actions are thus not interpreted as mistakes, but there is a defect in an organization's culture or value system if intentional wrongdoing is tolerated – that is, not discouraged and promptly sanctioned when it occurs.

Unavoidable mistakes

To promote organizational morale, the virtues of leaders may be excessively extolled and their shortcomings minimized or overlooked. Zero tolerance for mistakes may be self-imposed or promulgated by some senior executives – or, in the case of a CEO, perhaps by the governing body. To the extent this happens, executives do themselves a great disservice when they perpetuate unrealistic expectations.

Even the most capable executive will make mistakes. The effective healthcare executive will take calculated risks to develop innovative strategies and programs, recruit independent thinkers to the board and administrative staff, invest in new technology, respond to and shape the political and competitive environment, and challenge the status quo. Inevitably, an executive who is constantly considering different approaches and models will occasionally select a course that yields unanticipated and unwanted results.

In these less than successful situations, how extensive is the critique or failure analysis, and how broadly are the results disseminated? In actuality, the extent of analysis and disclosure is frequently limited because many executives may be reluctant to accept or admit the extent of their own fallibility. Defensively, they may also assert that insufficient time has passed to label a specific decision as "wrong." Consequently, mistakes are commonly hidden, like those of their clinical colleagues, behind what Smith and Forster (2000) describe as "a curtain of denial and nondisclosure." This curtain, however, is frequently transparent to subordinates and others. Furthermore, it is both ironic and disappointing that most programs dedicated to risk management and continuous quality improvement have essentially ignored such sensitive yet potentially fertile terrain.

Executives must be cautious not to take false refuge in the belief that a comprehensive and widely disseminated values statement is sufficient to ensure consistent adherence to those values. Few studies have been conducted to confirm an alignment between espoused organizational values and enacted values (Ray, Goodstein, and Garland 1999). Organizational culture and values have a powerful influence on the extent to which errors are recognized and analyzed. If the institution's vision and values statements promote the concept of a *learning organization* and the rhetoric is matched by reality, the positive aspects of individual pride and ego can contribute to an environment more open to unfettered inquiry and investigation of management as well as medical mistakes. In reality, very little learning occurs without making some mistakes.

Evolution of healthcare management mistakes

For at least the past four decades, so many publications have made repeated reference to the "healthcare crisis" that one may now reasonably contend that the crisis has become a chronic condition. The cumulative pressures produced by managed care, inadequate reimbursement, growing staff shortages, increasing competition, proliferating legal and regulatory requirements, rising expenses, higher patient and staff expectations, and a host of similar issues have conspired to make the difficulties seem overwhelming. Moreover, efforts to reduce overhead costs have resulted in fewer managers who have broader assignments and more subordinates. In addition, honoring the intrinsic obligation of a charitable institution to serve the community's best interest without adversely affecting the hospital's financial condition can create unusually complex management dilemmas (Vladeck 1992).

Contributing to the administrative challenge is the fact that healthcare executives have held less functional power than comparable managers in general business, primarily because physicians, who are generally not employees and hold an anomalous position outside the direct chain of command, exercise exceptional influence over management decisions. This imbalance of power can compel executives to make decisions that they personally find objectionable but that may be necessitated by the medical culture and accepted by the governing body. For example, at least some hospital-based physician contract terms could be difficult to defend on a productivity and service basis. In other situations, executives may have capitulated as the result of failing to engage physicians in a collaborative decision-making process. If physicians do not understand the inescapable resource constraints facing the institution and the need to help design a rational allocation system that preserves the organization's fiscal health, they may be inclined to adopt adversarial rather than cooperative approaches to resolving conflict.

Particularly in health systems, the need to make large financial turnarounds can create extensive organizational dissonance. If strategy, structure, process, and culture are not well aligned around a clear vision and mission, corporate administration and business units can be at odds. Not surprisingly, suspicion, resentment, and hostility will produce an unhealthy climate in which both management timidity and error can thrive. Mistrust, not administrative competency and innocence, is the dominant presumption. Consequently, some executives may be inclined to think more about avoiding risky decisions and less about making courageous ones. The challenge is intensified when clinical issues are involved.

To further exacerbate the problem, differentiating between a clinical mistake and a management error can be difficult; often they are inextricably intertwined. Also, some decisions are clearly errors, whereas others are simply immoral. The most obvious examples involve the familiar tension between financial and patient care priorities, for instance:

- Permitting early discharge of seriously ill patients because of economic pressures
- Closing a trauma center because too many patients lack insurance
- Reducing social work and home health personnel, with the result that patients are discharged without adequate regard for their ability to care for themselves
- Allowing an organ transplant program to continue for non-clinical reasons, although its volume is low and its patient outcomes are poor
- Using insufficiently trained lower-skilled personnel to perform duties previously assigned to higher-skilled and more expensive staff
- Deferring funding of essential but mundane capital equipment (replacement beds, sterilizers) to accommodate less urgent requests of influential physicians.

The reconciliation of tensions around resource allocation decisions, and the tradeoffs among them, cannot be avoided. Nor can the crucial link between cost and quality be ignored. However, improving quality does not always require more resources. In a hospital truly committed to a "patients first" philosophy, the above examples should not exist. Too frequently, management mistakes are repeated because previous assumptions about the tradeoffs between resource allocation decisions and quality are not subject to proper review, evaluation, and audit in the context of the institution's mission.

Many of the conflicts of interest that influence these decisions are apparent, but not all. Edward Spencer and his colleagues (2000) suggest that conflicts of interest occur in "situations where one's profession, professional judgment, or professional code is in conflict with other demands or influences that, if acted upon, would compromise professional judgment." The authors offer four guidelines when one is confronted with these circumstances:

(1) The existence of the conflict should be recognized and acknowledged
(2) Whenever possible, the conflict's existence should be disclosed to all parties
(3) A series of questions should be asked:
  (a) How would an impartial professional evaluate and act in this kind of situation?
  (b) Would acting on the conflict of interest compromise one's professional judgment?
  (c) What kinds of precedents would acting on this conflict set? Would you expect other professionals to act similarly? Can this be defended in a public forum?
  (d) Who is harmed or benefited from acting on the conflict of interest?
  (e) Can such actions prevent gratuitous harm or unfair practices, processes, or outcome; lying; breaking promises and contracts; and not respecting individuals and their rights?
  (f) What kind of institutional structure, accountability procedure, or other constraint might have contributed to the existence of this conflict? Can these factors be mitigated in the future?
(4) When encountering an unavoidable and intractable conflict of interest, one may have to withdraw from the situation and, in some circumstances, report the matter to an external entity.

Whether or not conflict of interest is a contributing factor, a decision may be made that could constitute a serious mistake and a "sentinel event." The Joint Commission on Accreditation of Healthcare Organizations (JCAHO 1999) defines a sentinel event as "an unexpected occurrence involving death or serious physical or psychological injury, or the risk thereof." When such an event occurs, JCAHO expects that "the organization will quickly, thoroughly, and credibly engage in a critical, self-reflective process known as root-cause analysis" (Johnson and Roebuck-Colgan 1999). Given that JCAHO's definition of a "sentinel event" is clinically focused, how might the concept be modified to accommodate an unexpected outcome due to an administrative decision? Is a root-cause analysis any less relevant in such a situation?

For the purposes of this discussion, I suggest the following definition of a sentinel event for use in stimulating a healthcare management internal investigation: *a sentinel administrative event is an unexpected occurrence involving major economic or non-economic losses adversely affecting patients or others or having the potential of leading to serious negative consequences.* Such an event is intended to include any significant development adversely affecting patients, the community, or financial or human resources. In these cases, conducting a root-cause analysis should be just as appropriate and potentially productive as when dealing with serious clinical problems.

At a minimum, such an analysis should attempt to identify the source of the error and its cause. First, to identify the source, a distinction should be made between a *manager's* mistake and a *management* mistake. This is not simply a semantic consideration; there is a substantive difference. A manager's decisions and actions, whether they are right or wrong, reflect how a particular individual manages her priorities, goals, values, and relationships. Most mistakes by managers are the result of mismanaging people and other resources, as well as inattention to critical details. In contrast to a manager's individual decisions and actions, management mistakes and successes usually result from collective decision-making. Poor systems will undermine the quality of decisions by both managers and management. Second, regardless of the source of the error, any informed analysis should include an examination of its cause(s). Table 1.1 includes a brief list of possible sources and causes of healthcare management mistakes.

Table 1.1   Sources and causes of healthcare management mistakes

Sources of mistakes
- Directed board decision
- Shared CEO/board decision
- CEO decision
- Shared CEO/management decision
- Shared CEO/medical staff or physician group decision
- Manager decision
- Shared manager/management decision

Causes of mistakes
- Inadequate preparation of/by decision-maker(s)
- Insufficient or inaccurate information
- Lack of expert input
- Ignorance of all legitimate alternatives
- Flawed decision-making process
- Carelessness
- Political pressure, fear, timidity
- Conflict of interest
- Undue haste
- Failure to follow established policies and/or external requirements

Management is subject to errors of omission as well as commission. Although errors of omission may be less apparent, their consequences can be just as damaging. Inaction or wrong decisions can occur because of (1) a personal preference for maintaining the status quo, (2) political pressure from internal or external stakeholders, (3) a failure to monitor the activities of subordinates, (4) becoming dependent on a need to support physicians' pecuniary interests, (5) excessive competitive drive or competitor emulation, (6) fear of making or admitting a mistake, (7) denial of the need to act, or (8) being personally over-extended physically, emotionally, or intellectually. A mistake can also be compounded by "escalating commitment," when efforts are redoubled in the belief that just trying harder will lead to success, rather than recognizing that the original idea or strategy was flawed. Table 1.2 lists errors of omission and commission.

Table 1.2   Errors of omission and commission

Omission
- Failure to anticipate significant factors affecting decisions
- Failure to act promptly on changed conditions
- Failure to consider all options
- Failure to delegate and hold subordinates accountable
- Failure to balance power interests
- Failure to keep patient and corporate needs paramount
- Failure to follow the law, economic principles, or the "prudent person" rule
- Failure to anticipate likely consequences
- Failure to fulfill contractual commitments and obligations to employees
- Failure to protect the assets of the corporation
- Failure to lead where there are opportunities to improve the health of patients or the community

Commission
- Permitting decisions to be made without adequate analysis
- Choosing political, not business solutions
- Making economic decisions that harm clinical care and outcomes
- Allocating limited resources without applying objective criteria
- Withholding negative information from individuals with the right to know
- Making selective use of facts with different audiences
- Showing favoritism among the board, management, medical staff, and employees
- Signing contracts that are not achievable
- Condoning discrimination among patient types on the basis of source of payment, ethnicity, gender, or other inappropriate or illegal factors
- Allowing a climate of male dominance to harm relationships between doctors and nurses, thus accelerating nurse turnover and poor patient care
- Making high-technology investments without addressing access problems

I must quickly note that not all acts of omission and commission necessarily constitute mistakes. The decision-maker may be limited to a small number of options, each of which has negative consequences. Likewise, the goals can be in conflict. For example, perhaps the only means of protecting the corporation's assets is to reduce or eliminate a vital community health program, as illustrated by the difficult choices faced by New York City's public hospital system (Steinhauer 2001). Thus, an economic choice could be made that reduces access to services, but every reasonable alternative may have been evaluated and dismissed as untenable. In other words, a "right" decision can still have bad results.

Management versus medical errors

In his book, *Forgive and Remember: Managing Medical Failure*, Bosk (1979) accurately observes that our healthcare institutions, like most organizations, rarely welcome questioning or admission of errors. The conspiracy of silence that once shielded many physicians has partially but not completely dissipated. Such a conspiracy also shields managers, and in some respects, management errors can be less obvious and perhaps more pernicious than those that occur in medicine.

Compared to medicine, defining error in management is even more difficult because perfection is especially elusive and standards of performance are poorly delineated. As suggested previously, management practices have far less precision, consensus, and objectivity than medical procedures. Formal processes and decision trees are not as prevalent in management as they are in medicine, resulting in fewer algorithms for enhancement. Consequently, there are many reasons, or perhaps excuses, for not pursuing a systematic analysis of management mistakes.

Although designed for medical errors, a proposed system by Smith and Forster (2000) also has relevance for examining management errors. They suggest a structure that (1) focuses on unintended acts only, leaving willful and malicious activity for other classifications and assessments; (2) includes "intercepted" mistakes without limiting identification of mistakes to a clear determination that a patient has been harmed by the mistake; (3) is not limited to a negligence standard (which focuses on legally culpable errors and is only a subset of all errors committed); (4) uses a skill-, rule-, and knowledge-based model as a mechanism to classify error types; and (5) provides a practical and reasonable standard for determining whether a mistake has occurred (e.g. an action that would have been judged wrong by skilled and knowledgeable peers at the time it occurred).

When a patient has been hurt or would have been severely harmed by an intercepted mistake, the consequences are clear. Because management errors may be more difficult to isolate, we should work diligently to find and apply any structure that promotes their timely disclosure.

Management science shares some other common characteristics with medical science. These include "inherent uncertainty, imperfect predictability, and unavoidable temporality" (Rubin and Zoloth 2000). But unlike medicine, in management there is little recognition of the need for programs encouraging prevention of mistakes, early detection, source determination, and timely correction. Although fewer management standards are available against which to measure performance, financial measures are plentiful (net income, credit rating, cash reserves, accounts receivable, debt ratio), as are those related to other outcomes influenced by healthcare management – for example, patient and staff satisfaction, staff turnover and vacancies, market share, institutional reputation, and, increasingly, quality and patient outcome measures.

Additional comparisons between medicine and management may provide further insights. Just as complexity, uncertainty, and imperfect information surround most medical encounters, making it difficult to define and categorize errors, the same is true of management mistakes. Decision-making errors in both medicine and management can be questionable or unverifiable. Also, as in medicine, mistakes in management may be the result of ignorance, negligence, or the inherently errant nature of the act. Regardless of the cause, there should be no "rush to judgment"; conclusions should not be drawn until the facts have been dispassionately evaluated.

Regrettably, medicine and management share another attribute that is not only destructive, but also underestimated in its influence on organizational and individual behavior. Abuse of power takes many forms and compromises anyone vulnerable to the improper exercise of authority or influence by another (Hofmann 1998). Whether the victims are patients, families, or staff, the degree and extent of intimidation can repress legitimate questioning of actions and decisions for an extended period. When such actions and decisions are wrong, the mistakes may not be revealed and, as a result, are often repeated.

Disclosure of management mistakes

Many management mistakes can be attributed to faulty information or data and can be reversed without causing substantial damage. Even those decisions that produce poor outcomes and that should not have occurred will benefit from disclosure and analysis. More serious are "reportable" mistakes involving an action with untoward results, the hiding or denial of which constitutes a breach of intellectual honesty or ethical behavior. These decisions should cause a conscientious person to have difficulty sleeping at night unless they are disclosed.

At a minimum, two levels of exposure should be considered in disclosing and preventing management mistakes. The first is the *macro* or policy level, at which the CEO, guided by the board, manages the organization's priorities, its relations with the outside world, and its strategic opportunities. At this level, at least initially, the CEO's ego and lack of objectivity may interfere with an ability to recognize and evaluate a major error, such as overextending financial and corporate resources in acquiring additional facilities. The second is the *micro* or operating level, at which the CEO establishes the institutional climate, makes decisions, and influences and monitors decisions made by others. However, at the micro level, there is less excuse for failing to acknowledge and disclose mistakes. Of course, the organization's culture and values predictably influence both levels.

Although executives should allow and encourage sincere disclosure of mistakes with impunity, they must not be hypocritical. For example, I recall an administrator who frequently urged his subordinates to give him constructive criticism and invariably responded defensively and somewhat belligerently when it was offered. As expected, despite his continuing reminders that he welcomed negative feedback, he rarely received it again. Executives who espouse the concept and then repudiate it by their reactions reflect a remarkable degree of arrogance at worst or naïveté at best. Ultimately, the question becomes: Is the organizational support real, or is it an ethical mirage?

Just as important as the timely disclosure of errors and a receptive climate is deciding to whom mistakes should be reported. Obviously, several factors must be evaluated, such as the magnitude of the error, the number of people compromised, if and when the mistake can be corrected, any mandated reporting requirements, implicit ethical obligations to disclose, and compliance with existing institutional policies. Generally, mistakes should be disclosed to those most affected by them and to those in authority – for example, the governing board. And yet, pragmatically, there are limits to the number of audiences to which disclosure is necessary. Unlimited candor is neither obligatory nor appropriate. If a hospital were to publicize every error, regardless of its size or consequences, the institution's reputation could be irreparably and unreasonably harmed. Because the least convenient time to develop any policy is in a time of crisis, organizations should establish disclosure criteria *in advance* of the need to apply them. Table 1.3 lists principal considerations for disclosure.

Fortunately, some positive signs about handling negative news have appeared. Noting the burden created by credit-rating agencies pursuing financial information, Carpenter (2001) has described the growing consensus among non-profit organizations that increased disclosure demonstrates a pattern of greater accountability and may actually result in a better reception for an issuer's bonds.

As clinicians and others promote a safer institutional environment for patients, families, and staff, what should executives do to promote more prudent management decisions in the future? Does the organizational culture encourage or

Table 1.3   Mistake disclosure considerations

What stimulus requires disclosure?	To whom should the error be disclosed?
Legally advised	Board
JCAHO required	Medical staff
Board mandated	Employees
Ethically determined	Media
	Community groups
Who should be the designated spokesperson?	**What other issues need to be taken into account?**
Board chair	Confidentiality and liability factors
CEO	Discussion of prevention measures
Legal counsel	
Public relations	

discourage candor and open discussion of management misjudgments? Does the organization recognize that truth telling and promise keeping are as relevant to business decisions as they are to clinical activity? Acknowledging the wisdom of the old adage to tell the truth early, when does *not* disclosing an error become indefensible?

The issues here are just as relevant to staff at all organizational levels as they are to the executive team. The economic and non-economic consequences of real or perceived cover-ups when mistakes do occur are undeniable. By encouraging timely and complete disclosure, organizations not only can act to minimize loss and exercise appropriate damage control, they also can move more quickly to learn from the mistake and strengthen or implement preventive measures.

Alternatively, discouraging disclosure by penalizing staff who report errors will promote a much less constructive activity – whistleblowing. Although frequently defined as an action taken when information is reported to an external organization about an allegedly illegal act or set of activities, whistleblowing can also include internal reporting of mistakes that may have been consciously suppressed by the person responsible for the error. Regardless of the circumstances, efforts to stifle timely disclosure are unethical. Darr (1997) notes that patients and families understand that mistakes will occur, but they cannot understand deceit. The same is no less true of staff members, who may know a management error has been made and resent attempts to conceal it.

Executives must realize that organizational dynamics will vary according to the type and magnitude of a mistake, as well as the stakeholders involved. The senior executive must take into account the following five core constituencies:

(1) *The board* – If the responsibility for a mistake is shared, the CEO will likely be held accountable for the consequences (and probably should be). Regardless of

who was responsible for the error, the CEO must decide if complete candor will be accepted by the board as part of properly addressing the problem or if unexpurgated disclosure will irreversibly compromise the executive's future influence. Non-disclosures or partial disclosures obviously carry their own risks.

(2) *Medical staff* – If a mistake is so serious that disclosure produces a vote of no confidence by the medical staff, the CEO will usually be forced to leave the organization. Depending on the CEO's tenure and reputation, timely disclosure of lesser mistakes may, in some situations, actually enhance the executive's credibility.

(3) *Management team* – Some mistakes will be the result of unilateral decisions and others will be the product of shared decision-making. In either case, disclosure and analysis usually contribute to team building and effectiveness. By discussing and dissecting the error, team members develop a better understanding of why the mistake occurred, how it might have been prevented, and how its harmful effects can be mitigated. Such an analysis also helps promote a constructive and non-punitive climate for revealing mistakes.

(4) *Employees* – Particularly if the mistake is "public knowledge," management should explain what happened, why it happened, and how the consequences will be addressed. There could be widely disparate interpretations of the decision, and one of the disclosure objectives is to sustain confidence in management.

(5) *Patients* – Medical errors, not management mistakes, are more likely to adversely affect patients and their families, but executives do make errors of commission and omission that affect individual patients and groups of patients, as illustrated previously.

The first of two other major constituencies, of course, is the community. Again, depending on the mistake and its relevance for the community, disclosure should be carefully evaluated. Factors to assess include confidentiality, legal obligations, current or potential harm to the community, liability exposure for the institution, and political repercussions. These same elements are pertinent to a second external group of constituents, namely regulators, payers, buyers, and vendors. Table 1.4 contains a broad taxonomy of management errors.

Coping with mistakes

Not all mistakes will or should produce feelings of embarrassment or guilt. But when an executive does have these feelings, how can they be assuaged? Should executives seek and receive forgiveness, and from whom? What should be the limits of personal and organizational loyalty? How can he or she deal with concerns about real or imagined liability?

Table 1.4   Typology of healthcare management error [a]

Levels	Classification
Macro (policy)	Economic
Micro (operational)	Organizational
	Strategic
	Clinical
Consequences	**Constituency influenced**
(Measured by number	The Board
of people and/or dollars	Medical staff
adversely affected)	Senior management
None	Employees
Moderate	Patients
Major	Community
	Regulators, payers, buyers, and vendors

Note: [a] None of these is mutually exclusive.

Like their clinical colleagues, some executives believe that they must be perfectionists. Most managers and physicians do not allow themselves the luxury of failure, and, consequently, they create a false sense of infallibility. Alternatively, rather than wanting to avert a mistake, their overriding concern may be taking the popular action and, as a result, not antagonizing or alienating an individual or a group. For example, it is much easier to avoid renegotiating untenable physician contracts than to deal with the ire of clinicians.

Given human nature, the level of embarrassment or guilt will vary depending on not whether but how much the executive rationalizes some degree of the error. Daigneault (1997), president of the Washington, DC-based Ethics Resource Center, has asked the question: "Why do good people do bad things?" Among the reasons, he cites are:

- a lack of organizational loyalty
- the way "success" is measured
- a belief that the act is not illegal
- the result of peer pressure.

In fact, as noted by Johnson and Roebuck-Colgan (1999): "A recurring theme in the literature about the process of root-cause analysis is that good people can be trapped in flawed systems." Blaming or being blamed is not constructive behavior, but dealing with guilt and even, in some situations, grief may still be necessary. Actually, the five stages encountered by many terminally ill patients – denial and shock, anger, bargaining, depression, and acceptance – may also be relevant in working through the analytical process (Kubler-Ross 1969). We must recognize which stage the decision-maker is in and how loyalty may have affected this person's attitude and actions.

Webster and Baylis (2000) say that moral distress can lead to compromised integrity and what they define as "moral residue." According to these authors, moral distress occurs "when there is incoherence between one's beliefs and one's actions, and possibly also outcomes (that is, between what one sincerely believes to be right, what one actually does, and what eventually transpires)." Moral distress does not occur just when institutional constraints make pursuing the right action difficult, but also when "one fails to pursue what one believes to be the right course of action (or fails to do so to one's satisfaction) for one or more of the following reasons: an error of judgment, some personal failing (for example, a weakness or crimp in one's character such as a pattern of 'systemic avoidance'), or other circumstances truly beyond one's control." Moral residue, they explain, "is that which each of us carries with us from those times in our lives when in the face of moral distress we have seriously compromised ourselves or allowed ourselves to be compromised." Among the reasons for doing so, they add, are expediency, laziness, and cowardice. In other words, sometimes it takes courage to choose the hard right over the easy wrong.

When a major management mistake is made, personal and organizational angst cannot always be avoided or eliminated. The imperative is to support those affected and to maintain a caring environment. According to Potter (1999), "When the captains of the industry understand the linkage among integrated bioethics, corporate integrity, and commercial success, there will be a rush to the moral bank for more social capital." This moral bank is in no current danger of being overdrawn.

If being a successful "transformational" business leader requires an individual who "blends extreme personal humility with intense professional will" (Collins 2001), acknowledging one's mistakes not only demonstrates fallibility, it also allows others the freedom to fail without fear of retribution. Andre (2000) describes why the virtue of humility is so central to an examination of errors:

On the one hand, mistakes are inevitable. On the other hand, they are to be avoided; nothing counts as a mistake unless in some sense we could have done otherwise. This fundamental paradox creates the moral challenge of accepting our fallibility and at the same time struggling against it. Humility is crucial to both aspects of this task – humility not of shame but of compassion toward oneself. At the heart of compassion is simple kindness, an attitude that is essential to clarity about oneself and to living with imperfection while striving mightily for something better.

Admitting, analyzing, and disclosing administrative errors should be considered legitimate dimensions of management maturity, but little evidence exists that such is the case.

What process should be followed by a CEO who has made a bad decision – one that, in retrospect, really was a serious error? Depending on the circumstances, coping with this mistake could involve some of the following steps.

(1) *Accept the truth* by documenting the problem, its roots, and its consequences, and include options for addressing the mistake. If appropriate, solicit advice from peers or a consultant.

(2) *Speak with selected officers* of the board, medical staff, management, and/or legal counsel.

(3) Present a *summary* to the management team and facilitate a discussion and analysis.

(4) Determine if a *new policy or refinement of an existing policy* would minimize the repetition of a similar error.

(5) Decide if the organization's supervisory development program or any other training activities should incorporate insights acquired as the result of this process.

Clarifying the limits of personal and organizational loyalty can be helpful to both the individual and the institution. Occasionally out of personal loyalty, but more often due to a concern about retribution and a fear of the consequences, subordinates may be reluctant to report a manager's mistake either to that individual or the person at the next management level. The disclosure is even more problematic if the CEO has made the error and there is evidence that it has not been disclosed immediately to the board.

Assuming that the mistake does not justify termination, a supportive organization will provide for a thorough examination of the error, not with the goal of placing blame, but for the purpose of identifying problems and learning from the experience. Circumstances will determine whether an apology should be offered, and to whom. As in personal relationships, too seldom are there expressions of regret that can defuse emotions and permit mutual healing to occur. Similarly, in some situations, simply seeking forgiveness will not be enough; arrangements for making amends should also be made.

Undeniably, occasions will arise when the gravity of the mistake or combination of mistakes justifies discharging or disciplining a manager. Most organizations want to avoid taking this action and, even when warranted, may delay moving expediently. In some situations, the individual could be impaired by psychological problems or substance abuse; in other cases, the person may have been promoted beyond her level of competency. Procrastination usually serves neither the organization nor the manager well. Regardless of the circumstances, the proper board or management response will reflect sensitivity for the individual and the organization.

In a highly litigious society, the possibility of legal liability should obviously not be ignored. Again, depending on the nature of the mistake, the potential exposure may be real or imagined. Damages quickly escalate when there is proof that the action was an avoidable flaw, for example, "up-coding" or other evidence of overbilling. Healthcare institutions, like other businesses, must be vigilant in their dissemination and enforcement of policies mandating compliance with local, state, and federal laws and regulations. The combination of the 1991 Federal Sentencing Commission guidelines and the 1996 Health Insurance Portability and Accountability Act has made compliance an unprecedented priority, but as Paine (1994) has observed, "managers who define ethics as legal compliance are implicitly endorsing a code of moral mediocrity for their organizations." Orientation and continuing education programs represent convenient opportunities to convey an unambiguous message to both supervisory and non-supervisory staff that the spirit as well as the letter of these requirements must be met.

Improving management performance

To risk stating the obvious, competent management involves much more than preventing or morally managing mistakes. Challenging times demand aggressive and innovative leadership, not risk-averse executives who are hesitant to make difficult decisions. We should be examining our informal decision systems and assessing how their ambiguity may contribute to uneven management outcomes. The unacceptable alternative is to rationalize our inability to emulate our clinical colleagues who continue to refine their decision-making processes and achieve more consistent and predictable results. Hopefully, just as evidence-based medicine has contributed significantly to improving clinical decisions, the belated emergence of evidence-based management in healthcare may eventually have the same salutary impact on administrative decisions (Kovner, Elton, and Billings 2000; Walshe and Rundall 2001).

Ethically, making a mistake haphazardly or cavalierly is vastly different from making one using formally designed decision-making processes that are rigorous, open, and rational. If an error occurs as the result of a logical disciplined process, it is still unfortunate, but one's ethical "liability" is limited. Worthley (1999) contends that a mature ethical reasoning process is characterized by collaboration and a systematic methodology. In contrast, he says that a single-minded ethical reasoning process "inevitably degenerates and debilitates judgment."

To enhance ethical reasoning when making a decision, Nash (1981) suggests that twelve questions should be raised to maximize an understanding of the responsibilities involved and to promote the decision-maker's objectivity:

(1) Have you defined the problem *accurately*?

(2) How would you define the problem if you stood on the *other* side of the fence?

(3) *How* did this situation occur in the first place?

(4) To whom and to what do you give your *loyalty*, as a person and as a member of the corporation?

(5) What is your *intention* in making this decision?

(6) How does this intention compare with the probable *results*?

(7) Whom could your decision or action *injure*?

(8) Can you *discuss* the problem with the affected parties before you make your decision?

(9) Are you confident that your position will be as *valid* over a long period of time as it seems now?

(10) Could you *disclose* without qualm your decision or action to your boss, your CEO, the board of directors, your family, or society as whole?

(11) What is the *symbolic potential* of your action if understood? If misunderstood?

(12) Under what conditions would you allow *exceptions* to your stand?

A specific process or methodology does not guarantee an ethically defensible outcome, but Worthley (1997) indicates that it "can help healthcare professionals identify and utilize the resources needed to advance ethical maturity." At a minimum, executives have a responsibility to ensure that simple systems are implemented to prevent, discourage, detect, and address mistakes.

A modest beginning might involve a decision system that promotes the prevention of management errors, minimizes bad decisions at the outset, discloses and addresses mistakes afterwards, and conveys a clear message that examining and understanding the reasons for mistakes represents a learning opportunity. Such a system would:

- Be designed with clear *objectives, formal criteria, and explicit performance measures;* reflect relevant organizational values and policies; and incorporate a process that sensitizes the decision-maker to the implications for affected stakeholders.
- Provide for *decision tracking and evaluation*, including (a) programs to encourage the "safe" disclosure of problems and (b) error detection through an audit procedure that defines accountability, outcome measures, and timelines.
- Require a *post-implementation analysis* to explore factors that may have contributed to flaws in the original decision-making process.
- Specify a range of options to *minimize the immediate effect of future errors*, including both economic and non-economic costs, as well as possible longer-term organizational impact.
- Designate what actions will be considered to prevent similar mistakes in the future, including *revisions in policies, procedures, and business practices.*

Any such system will not function effectively unless the organization's CEO and governing body are unequivocally committed to establishing and sustaining a climate conducive to reducing management errors. According to Cashman (1999), CEO leadership requires three elements. The first is *authenticity* – is the person believable, real, humble? The second is *self-expression* – can the CEO communicate the institution's vision in language relevant to the staff? And the third is *value* – does the leader bring real benefit in terms of the bottom line, quality, and improved performance? Each of these elements is vital to promoting a culture that not only permits but also encourages the timely identification, disclosure, and resolution of management errors.

Recommendations

Although management mistakes will certainly continue to occur, a number of steps can be taken to increase the probability that they will be managed appropriately:

(1) Health administration programs should make use of *case studies* and *presentations* by executives to promote discussion of the problems and opportunities created by errors.

(2) *National bodies*, such as the American College of Healthcare Executives, American Hospital Association (AHA), Catholic Health Association, Premier, Veterans Administration, and VHA should explore their possible roles in helping healthcare leaders implement procedures to reduce management mistakes.

(3) *Organizational and professional codes of ethics* should be followed and monitored, but they are not a panacea and their limitations should be recognized (Brien 1996; Higgins 2000).

(4) The *rhetoric of a learning organization* should be aligned with reality by:

  (a) Emphasizing the institution's philosophy and values regarding both management and clinical mistakes in orientation and continuing education programs.

  (b) Using a management retreat to summarize a current management dilemma, highlight competing interests, and raise critical questions. The participants should be stimulated to develop new insights and be better prepared for existing and subsequent challenges. As described by Reiser (1994): "Cases illuminating the relationships and actions of organizations can be used to: test how effectively the values in institutional statements of purpose are applied in practice; formulate and critique policies and goals; analyze troublesome problems; and create an institutional memory to guide future policies."

  (c) Including several questions or statements to assess employee perceptions in regularly scheduled opinion and attitude surveys. For example:

- Does the organization allow, within reasonable limits, the administrative freedom to fail, or is the fear of potential criticism so great that managers rarely exercise initiative?
- Do individuals feel comfortable disclosing management mistakes? What will these individuals do if certain errors are made? What have they done in the past?
- Are identifiable resources available to provide constructive advice when mistakes are made? Who can staff members consult if they are uncertain what to do?
- Is there an external entity to whom they can go if internal lines are blocked?
- Have respondents encountered retribution when mistakes have been reported or disclosed?

(d) Conducting an organizational ethics audit to determine gaps between formal policies and actual behavior. Such an audit would not only incorporate an inventory of existing documents, but also training programs, committees, challenges facing the institution, and staff perceptions of the organization's ethics standards and practices (AHA 1997). Most management mistakes are *not* ethical ones; however, policies on advertising, receipt of gifts, confidentiality, sexual harassment, and uncompensated care do have ethical implications, as do the organization's vision, mission, and values statements.

(5) CEOs should establish a predetermined date and allocate time, as part of a strategic investment decision-making process, to assess whether the results have met forecasted *outcomes*. Time is always in short supply, but somehow adequate time is found when litigation occurs in response to a major error.

(6) *Annual CEO performance reviews* should be modified to incorporate questions or statements promoting discussion of mistakes and how they were addressed. At the senior management level, pivotal issues would include the outcomes of strategic initiatives involving the medical staff as well as the board; responses and non-responses to competitive market forces, health plans, and reimbursement changes; significant budget variances; staffing shortages; and indigent care. The self-assessment component should provide reflections about decisions that, in retrospect, were incorrect or inappropriate. In addition, the governing body's own annual self-assessment process should include a review of its role in learning about mistakes and evaluating them.

(7) *Supervisory performance reviews* should also include how the individual has dealt with her mistakes and the individual's response to the mistakes of others.

Has there been a tendency to shift blame or to accept and promote account-ability (Friedman 2001)?

(8) CEOs should develop a *policy governing management mistakes* and submit it to their boards for consideration. The development and discussion of policies and guidelines can help employees at all levels understand the limits of personal and organizational loyalty and decide how to proceed when con-fronted with a substantive management mistake. When a direct approach is not viewed as safe or productive, the individual might seek advice from a colleague, use a telephone hot line, consult with someone in human resources (HR), or take another step described in the guidelines. Table 1.5 lists the components that should be covered in a policy on management mistakes. This document should be written in simple language appropriate for employees and distributed to all staff members. (An alternative would

Table 1.5   Components for a policy on management mistakes

Preface	Includes the policy's purpose and describes the importance of identifying, confirming, investigating, reporting, and addressing management mistakes
Definition of management mistake	Provides a definition created by the organization reflecting its specific culture, values, and expectations; includes hypothetical examples or even actual mistakes from the organization's history
Criteria for reporting mistakes	Establishes criteria for bringing alleged mistakes to the attention of appropriate individuals
Assurance of non-recrimination	Assures staff members that recriminations against reporting staff members will not be permitted or tolerated
Disclosure of mistakes	Reviews the organization's process for determining to whom mistakes will be disclosed
Description of available resources	Describes the roles of administration, human resources, legal counsel, risk management, compliance office, ethics committee, and other resources in addressing management mistakes
Summary of procedures	Explains what steps should be taken when a reportable mistake has occurred

be the development of a policy on management decision-making that incorporates elements of both the decision system described previously and components of the policy on management mistakes.)

(9) Executives should serve as *role models and mentors* to demonstrate how to behave ethically. They can encourage others to do so by following Dye's (2000) admonitions to: (a) tell the truth and not exaggerate, (b) ensure that actions match words, (c) use power appropriately, and (d) admit mistakes.

(10) *Ethics committees* should expand their role beyond the traditional focus on clinical matters (Seeley and Goldberger 1999). Whether described as management, organizational, institutional, or business ethics, the related issues have much in common with clinical ethics.

Conclusion

Devoting appropriate attention to management mistakes requires a board that is truly deliberative and well informed – one that has created a relationship with its CEO based on mutual trust and confidence as well as respect. Also required are management staff members who are challenged by the CEO to be loyal skeptics, not simply unquestioning followers. Such an attitude is encouraged and supported when supervisors are motivated to express their views about dubious projects and to acknowledge their own mistakes. Finally, this climate must be sustained by (1) internal systems producing accurate and timely information that is widely available, (2) formal training programs across the organization on how to use information effectively, and (3) a culture that listens and responds.

Executives cannot avoid making mistakes. The repercussions from unintentional errors will range from negligible to enormous. To manage them properly, it is imperative that they be defined, disclosed, and analyzed, their economic and non-economic consequences be understood, and their recurrence be minimized. Many mistakes by managers might be prevented or mitigated by less hubris and more willingness to seek advice and obtain further input. In the absence of incentives to acknowledge and examine management mistakes, individual and organizational integrity will be damaged. More importantly, patients, family members, staff, and the community served by the institution will be compromised.

Denial and rationalization are convenient forms of ethical amnesia. Acknowledging and addressing management mistakes requires that executives admit their fallibility and promote an organizational environment that makes it safe to report and evaluate our imperfections.

The journey is not an easy or simple one. Not all executives will be able to transform their management style to accommodate the personal growth required. The most effective leader will be one who thinks in terms of change and renewal, not merely survival; is a coach and facilitator, not an autocrat; focuses on quality and service, not just the bottom line; builds commitment rather than demanding compliance; and empowers people instead of controlling them. The trip should therefore not be undertaken without a full appreciation of the challenges that will be encountered but knowing that the potential benefits are incalculable.

REFERENCES

American Hospital Association, 1997. *AHA's Organizational Ethics Initiative.* Chicago: American Hospital Association

Andre, J., 2000. "Humility reconsidered," in S. B. Rubin and L. Zoloth (eds.). *Margin of Error: The Ethics of Mistakes in the Practice of Medicine.* Hagerstown, MD: University Publishing

Bosk, C., 1979. *Forgive and Remember: Managing Medical Failure.* Chicago: University of Chicago Press

Brien, A., 1996. "Regulating virtue: formulating, engendering and enforcing corporate ethics codes." *Business and Professional Ethics Journal* **15(1)**: 21–52

Carpenter, D., 2001. "Filling the information gap." *Investor Relations, A Supplement to Health Forum Journal* **44:(3)**: 4–8

Cashman, K., 1999. *Leadership from the Inside Out: Becoming a Leader for Life.* Provo, UT: Executive Excellence Publishing

Collins, J., 2001. "Level 5 leadership: the triumph of humility and fierce resolve." *Harvard Business Review* **79(1)**: 66–76

Costello, M., 2000. "Early '90s merger mania gives over to 'divorce court.'" *AHA News* **36(15)**: 2

Daigneault, M., 1997. "Why Ethics?" *Association Management* **49(9)**: 28–34

Darr, K., 1997. *Ethics in Health Services Management.*, Baltimore, MD: Health Professions Press

Dye, C. F., 2000. *Leadership in Healthcare: Values at the Top.* Chicago: Health Administration Press

Friedman, E., 2001. "The butler did it." *Healthcare Forum Journal* **44(4)**: 5–7

Garvin, D. A., 2000. *Learning in Action: A Guide to Putting the Learning Organization to Work.* Boston: Harvard Business School Press

Greenspan, B., 2002. "Protecting the Community's Trust: Coping with Executive Mistakes." *Frontiers of Health Services Management* **18(3)**: 35–40

Higgins, W., 2000. "Ethical guidance in the era of managed care: an analysis of the American College of Healthcare Executives." *Journal of Healthcare Management* **45(1)**: 32–34

Hilfiker, D. 1984. "Facing Our Mistakes." *New England Journal of Medicine* **310**: 118–122

Hofmann, P. B., 1991. "Hospitals eroding public trust." *Modern Healthcare* **21(37)**: 20
    1998. "Abuse of power." *Healthcare Executive* **14(2)**: 55–56

Joint Commission on Accreditation of Healthcare Organizations (JCAHO), 1999. *Comprehensive Accreditation Manual for Hospitals*, secs. AC.6 and PI.4.3. Oakbrook Terrace, IL: Joint Commission on Accreditation of Healthcare Organizations

Johnson, K. M. and K. Roebuck-Colgan, 1999. "Organizational ethics and sentinel events: doing the right thing when the worst thing happens." *The Journal of Clinical Ethics* **10(3)**: 237–241

Institute of Medicine, 1999. *To Err is Human: Building a Safer Health System*. Washington, DC: Institute of Medicine and National Academy Press.

Kovner, A. R., J. L. Elton, and J. Billings, 2000. "Evidence-based management." *Frontiers of Health Services Management* **16(2)**: 3–24

Kubler-Ross, E., 1969. *On Death and Dying*. New York: Simon & Schuster

Nash, L., 1981. "Ethics without the sermon." *Harvard Business Review* **59(6)**: 79–90

Paine, L., 1994. "Managing for organizational integrity." *Harvard Business Review* **72(2)**: 106–118

Potter, R. L., 1999. "On our way to integrated bioethics: clinical/organizational/communal." *The Journal of Clinical Ethics* **10(3)**: 171–177

Ray, L. N., J. Goodstein and M. Garland, 1999. "Linking professional and economic values in healthcare organizations." *The Journal of Clinical Ethics* **10(3)**: 216–223

Reiser, S. J., 1994. "The ethical life of healthcare organizations." *Hastings Center Report* **24(6)**: 28–35

Russell, S., 2000. "$176 million tab on failed hospital merger." *San Francisco Chronicle* December 14

Rubin, S. B. and L. Zoloth. 2000. "Introduction: in the margins of the margin." in S. B. Rubin and L. Zoloth (eds.), *Margin of Error: The Ethics of Mistakes in the Practice of Medicine* Hagerstown, MD: University Publishing.

Seeley, C. R. and S. L. Goldberger, 1999. "Integrated ethics: synecdoche in healthcare." *The Journal of Clinical Ethics* **10(3)**: 202–209

Smith, M. and H. Forster, 2000. "Morally managing medical mistakes." *Cambridge Quarterly of Healthcare Ethics* **9(1)**: 38–53

Spencer, E. M., A .E. Mills, M. V. Rorty, and P. H. Werhane, 2000. *Organization Ethics in Health Care*. New York: Oxford University Press

Steinhauer, J., 2001. "After 5 years of fiscal success, city public hospitals face deficit." *The New York Times* May 23

Vladeck, B. 1992. "Healthcare leadership in the public interest." *Frontiers of Health Services Management* **8(3)**: 3–26

Walshe, K. and T. G. Rundall, 2001. "Evidence-based management: from theory to practice in healthcare." *The Milbank Quarterly* **79(3)**: 429–457

Webster, G. C. and F. E. Baylis, 2000. "Moral residue," In S. B. Rubin and L. Zoloth (eds.), *Margin of Error: The Ethics of Mistakes in the Practice of Medicine* Hagerstown, MD: University Publishing

Worthley, J. A., 1997. *The Ethics of the Ordinary in Healthcare: Concepts and Cases*. Chicago: Health Administration Press

1999. *Organizational Ethics in the Compliance Context*. Chicago: Health Administration Press

2

The context of managerial mistakes

John Abbott Worthley

Despite our best efforts and self-image of high competence, we do all make mistakes. At executive levels in healthcare this reality is no less true than it is in business, in academia, in church organizations, or in the military. The CEO of American Airlines and many others in business, the president of St. Bonaventure University, numerous Catholic bishops, and the heads of both the Air Force and Naval Academies have been visible examples in 2003 alone. Recent indictments of healthcare executives with the Tenet Corporation and other healthcare institutions are receiving considerable notoriety as well (Abelson 2003).

To better understand the reality and position ourselves to turn the phenomenon of mistakes in a managerially helpful direction, some illumination of the context in which management mistakes unfold is important. This chapter is designed to do just that. Some of the context is generic – common to all organizational settings; some of the context is specific to healthcare entities. For conceptual clarity we explore the context by distinguishing eight major aspects: legal, organizational, financial, political, professional, ethical, social and psychological.

Legal dimensions

Probably the most obvious dimension of the context of managerial mistakes is the legal aspect. It is rather visible, and mistakes in this area can have serious consequences for the individual executive and for the corporation. Prison time and significant fines, as well as negative publicity and reduced market performance, are part of the reality. The plethora of corporate and contractual statutes constitutes a foundation upon which is built a maze of legal and procedural standards for all organizations. Failures to follow the law are, of course, major mistakes that can ruin careers, endanger clients,

Management Mistakes in Healthcare, ed. Paul Hofmann and Frankie Perry. Published by Cambridge University Press. © Cambridge University Press 2005.

and jeopardize organizational viability. Medical malpractice is also a major aspect, encompassing as it does both clinical and managerial liability for mistakes.

In healthcare the legal dimension includes a panoply of laws, rules, and procedures that condition nearly every aspect of healthcare work from operational, financial and procedural matters to research, transplants, and most clinical activities. Major legislation, such as the Health Insurance Portability and Accountability Act (HIPAA) and the 2002 Sarbanes–Oxley Act, is the most significant addition to this legal dimension.

HIPAA was enacted in 1996 to govern privacy, security, and electronic transactions standards for personal information. It became effective in healthcare in 2001 and provides stiff penalties (up to ten years in prison and fines of $250,000) for mistakes in managing personal healthcare information. The Sarbanes–Oxley Act responds to the recent corporate accounting scandals and establishes rigorous managerial responsibility for financial disclosure.

Because consequences can be so severe and public the legal context has been relatively well attended to. Healthcare organizations have learned to pay high attention and spend billions on legal counsel, training, detailed policies and procedures, and other means of ensuring that this context is well monitored so that legal mistakes are minimized.

Overarching the legal context in healthcare is the development of "compliance." Beginning in 1991, the Federal Sentencing Commission issued guidelines that have resulted in the concept of "compliance" becoming one of the most recognized and "buzzword" notions in corporate America, including healthcare (Worthley 1999). The movement began as a straightforward effort to establish uniformity in penalties given to offenders against federal law and regulations. However, as the movement evolved, the Commission embraced a creative approach using the old "carrot and stick" analogy. The "stick" would be very significant monetary fines and prison terms for mistakes involving federal standards. It includes a *qui tam* provision whereby investigators encourage whistleblowing by offering a percentage of any eventual fine. The "carrot" aspect provides for major leniency in penalties for mistakes if the organization has in place a rigorous compliance programe i.e. an organizational process for preventing, detecting, and reporting mistakes. Because of the considerable economic incentive, most healthcare organizations have established such compliance programs (Gunn, Goldfarb, and Showalter 1998). Furthermore, judges have been consistent in basing the degree of leniency on the extent of pre-existing organizational efforts.

The compliance aspect of the legal dimension, thus, realistically expects that mistakes will occur and therefore attempts to create a legal atmosphere which encourages and rewards efforts to minimize mistakes, to monitor and report their occurrence, and to act responsibly when mistakes come to light. This legal dimension of the context of managerial mistakes, while huge and complicated, is a positive and helpful reality for executives working to deal with and learn from the phenomenon of management mistakes.

Organizational dimensions

Managerial mistakes obviously take place within organizations. The context, therefore, has both formal/structural organizational elements as well as informal/ cultural organizational elements. Since mistakes are usually a function of both the individual and the environment, the nature of the organizational setting and its effect on mistakes (whether facilitating them or minimizing them) is of considerable importance in addressing the phenomenon.

A simple matrix (Table 2.1) can be helpful in comprehending the organizational context. The matrix provides a sort of lens through which to better see and analyze the organizational context.

The official, and fairly obvious, aspect of organizations – typically termed the "formal organization" – refers to structural realities such as organization charts and written policies. The much less obvious realities, such as grapevines and unwritten policies, are usually termed organizational culture or "informal organization." The formal structure concerns what presumably *should* characterize organizational life; the informal culture concerns what *actually* characterizes organizational life. Of course, a close interaction exists between the two, and each affects the other. The relevant question is: Do these formal and informal realities encourage or help to minimize managerial mistakes?

An analogy to highway driving might help us discern. Formally, there are in place official speed limits, radar equipment, and laws governing traffic violations. Do these encourage or reduce driving mistakes? Perhaps if speed limits, for example, are set too low they might actually facilitate driving mistakes such as dangerous passing. Culturally, many drivers travel a bit above official speed limits and often police officers, for practical reasons, set their radar gauges above the official limit. Traffic safety agencies continue to seek effective ways to reduce driving mistakes by both adjusting formal structures and by direct efforts to adjust attitudes, customs, and other "cultural" aspects of driving.

Table 2.1   The organizational context

	Corporate	Group	Individual
Formal realities			
Informal realities			

So too, to affect the mistake phenomenon in healthcare organizations, we need to reflect on analogous realities and seek effective ways to facilitate mistake reduction. This requires reflection on the nature of our organization, which entails analysis of both formal structures and informal patterns. For example, we have in place extensive formal protocols to contain healthcare costs. In addition, clinical guidelines, referral requirements, and quality assurance programs are standard in healthcare today. Do these organizational structures encourage or reduce medical and financial mistakes? Informally, do physicians find ways to order expensive tests because of malpractice fears and organizational pressures to utilize equipment? Or do these structures result in misdiagnoses because of inadequate testing?

Both formal and cultural realities of organizations can be more readily explored by recognizing – as the matrix suggests – that each consists of a corporate, group, and individual dimension. Each element interacts with and impacts the others. Using this construct, six elements can be identified for exploring the organizational context of managerial mistakes: formal corporate realities, informal corporate realities, formal group realities, informal group realities, formal individual realities, and informal individual realities.

By isolating each of these elements, we can focus on how the realities do and could facilitate or impede managerial mistakes. For each element, we can identify specific *structures* and *behaviors* and then think through whether they are a positive or a negative factor in terms of managerial mistakes. At the formal corporate level, for example, we can look at policies, codes, authority structure, department and committee structure, procedures, and systems of control, monitoring, and evaluation. At the formal group level, we can look at work group structures and relationships, group tasks, and local group procedures; at the formal individual level, job descriptions, performance evaluations, degree of isolation or interaction, and training programs can be examined. Each of these elements can be explored in terms of whether, and how, they contribute to the avoidance or commitment of managerial mistakes, and how they might be modified.

Another helpful concept for clarifying the organizational context of managerial mistakes is the "before–during–after" construct:

- What does the organization do structurally *before* mistakes are made? Does it plan avoidance strategies and tactics?
- What does the organization do structurally *during* mistake-making? Does it monitor for mistakes?
- What does the organization do structurally *after* mistakes are discovered? Does it report, analyze, and use them as input for bettering mistake prevention efforts?

These questions about structure need to be augmented by questions about cultural realities and their relationship to management mistakes. The informal cultural reality is much more subtle than the formal structural realities. It is unofficial and undocumented but extremely influential on organizational beha-vior. A key part of analysis of the organizational context of management mistakes is discernment of consistency, or lack thereof, between what is *formally stated and established* and what is *actually understood and done*.

The informal realities include elements such as power, norms, patterns, social groups, stress levels, pressure, feelings, and attitudes. Their importance in the mistake-making context is highlighted in a recent study that found that American corporations experience a high level of pressure to act inappropriately (Petry, Mujica, and Vickery 1998). Healthcare organizations, perhaps owing to financial challenges, reported among the highest levels of such informal pressure. This study found that the most frequently discovered mistakes involved the cutting of corners on quality control, falsifying reports, covering-up incidents, deceiving clients, withholding information, and misusing corporate property. In all cases, the study found, the formal organization had sound structures in place for preventing these mistakes while the informal organization had elements that actually encour-aged the kinds of mistakes committed. In other words, there was a significant inconsistency between formal and cultural realities. Factors identified as causing the inconsistencies included poor internal communications, inordinate emphasis on financial success, and market competition.

Leadership is an overarching key. The way leaders think, operate, coach, and analyze sends unmistakable signals about matters such as cutting corners, telling the truth, and the like. Inconsistency in these functions breeds mistakes. The questions leaders ask or neglect to ask, their responses to ideas, and their reaction to problems set a tone that facilitates or impedes mistakes. This is leadership. For example, I was recently present in a hospital setting when a speech therapist approached an elderly patient for an initial evaluation, called her by her first name, and proceeded to analyze her stroke/speech impairment with an unintended but unmistakably condescending tone. By chance, in the midst of this, the hospital CEO – who makes a practice of visiting ten patients a month – entered the room. He addressed the patient as "Mrs. H" and in a humble and respective tone asked if things were going well. The impact on those present far exceeded the impact of formal directives to treat patients with dignity. This was leadership in action. In effect, the informal power or influence of managers may be significantly more influential on the mistake phenomenon than their formal authority. Clearly the organizational context is an important aspect of management mistake-making.

Financial dimensions

Money, not surprisingly, is often a factor in management mistake-making. Financial fears and pressures are powerful forces and can be blinders to clear

Table 2.2   The financial context

	Corporate	Group	Individual
Formal financial structures *Informal financial culture*			

thinking. The matrix used to explore the organizational context above can be helpful in this dimension as well. The financial context includes corporate, group, and individual realities at both formal and cultural levels, as the matrix in Table 2.2 suggests.

At the formal financial level reward systems, such as compensation and promotion, usually emphasize financial performance in concert with many other performance factors. But informally, market competition, board pressure, and subtle supervisory signals often make it clear that financial success is primary. This in turn can create a corporate culture that, in effect, encourages mistakes such as cutting corners, offering inappropriate favors, and "fudging" numbers – the kinds of misguided organizational behaviors that have excited the media in recent years.

At the formal group level, units, departments, and work teams typically have fairly precise standards and procedures for operational activities. But informally, competitiveness can provoke a "group think" in which efforts to make the group look good result in using financial resources in questionable ways. Team playing can then engender a taboo about even questioning such dubious practices, making mistakes even more likely.

Group spirit and cohesiveness has also been known to result in financial rewards being given to members who are simply "team players," their actual performance notwithstanding.

At the formal individual level, job descriptions, codes of ethics, performance assessment instruments, and so forth usually establish an array of standards for individual behavior. But again, informally, reality may overemphasize financial performance, leading to improper behaviors. Formally, for example, most individual managers whom I know bring to the job a laudable sense of integrity and ethics. Informally, however, job insecurity, desire for bonuses, competitive spirit and the like have led to mistaken individual efforts to focus on financial outcome tactics which in turn have led to actions such as "cooking the books." So often even terrible mistakes are hardly about bad people making bad decisions; rather they are about mistaken perceptions by good people.

The financial reality that confronts healthcare organizations today clearly establishes a context of financial pressure that can readily facilitate management mistakes. Attention is therefore essential if such mistakes are to be minimized.

Political dimensions

Our simple matrix can also be usefully employed to uncover a political context for management mistakes. The notion of "office politics" has evolved, after all, from real-world experience, not from academic theorizing. It is instructive to isolate both formal and informal political realities at corporate, group and individual levels and to probe their effect on the management-mistake phenomenon (Table 2.3).

At the formal corporate level, for example, the typical healthcare organization has policies, codes, and procedures designed to prohibit "political" behavior such as preferential treatment and favoritism in customer relations as well as employment practices. But, informally, subtle counter pressures can often arise. When, for example, a corporate benefactor needs a corporate favor, ways are sometimes found to bend or waive standards and procedures so that such political interests can be accommodated. When a physician who is key to generating hospital admissions favors certain corporate directions, he or she may well exert considerable political pressure. At the group level, again, formal standards and procedures usually highlight fairness and neutrality in operations and official relationships; but, informally, normal social relationships are bound to exist and to exert some significant inclinations toward mistaken favoritism. The term "office politics" is reflective of this reality. When it comes to analysis of management mistakes, it does matter when people with whom I dine and play golf are involved in my management decisions and actions.

Even at the individual level, it is useful to evaluate the political context in terms of impact on management mistakes. Formally, of course, my political party affiliation and personal ideology should not affect my decisions. Informally, however, might my personal views on abortion, for example, tend to taint my performance assessment of an employee I know to have undergone an abortion? Hopefully not, but contextual analysis of management mistakes would not simply ignore the possibility. Let us also not fail to recognize the political clout that a major vendor can exercise. The analytical question, of course, is whether these undeniable political realities influence the mistake phenomenon positively or negatively.

Table 2.3   The political context

	Corporate	Group	Individual
Formal political structures			
Informal political realities			

Politics is a healthy and normal reality of everyday human life, including organizational life. It forms part of the context in which management mistakes occur or are prevented. Attention to its real influences is warranted.

Professional dimensions

It may be helpful to distinguish a professional context when analyzing the phenomenon of mistakes. Most healthcare managers participate in a professional society such as the American College of Healthcare Executives (ACHE) or the American Hospital Association (AHA). Formally, these organizations exert influences that may well temper mistake-making. They promulgate and espouse codes of conduct, they publish various reminders on good management practices, and they convene conferences and training programs aimed at facilitating exemplary management.

Informally, these same societies help to develop networks of healthcare managers that, in turn, sometimes engender "old boy network" behaviors that have been known to impair judgment and to facilitate mistake-making. While formally establishing and promoting standards designed to minimize mistakes, informally, professional identity and *esprit de corps* can also produce the "blue wall of silence" syndrome in which professional colleagues mistakenly protect managers known to be mistake-prone. When either professional or personal loyalty trumps proper organizational standards, management mistakes can emerge.

Efforts to better manage the mistake phenomenon can clearly benefit from strategic use of the formalities of the professional context as well as from careful scrutiny of the informalities. A particularly important aspect of this context unique to healthcare management is the Joint Commission for the Accreditation of Healthcare Organizations (JCAHO), the professional accrediting agency that formally sets standards largely designed to minimize mistake-making in healthcare delivery. The formal process of JCAHO monitoring, auditing, and reporting can obviously be a great help in reducing management mistakes. On the other hand, because of the competitive nature of the healthcare industry today, JCAHO audit results have significant marketplace implications and can, consequently, exert subtle influence on managerial judgment. High ratings are organizationally advantageous while low ratings are deleterious to the organization. Naturally, managers pay close attention to the JCAHO process. Informally, this tends to create a pressure to do well when the JCAHO team evaluates the organization. While this pressure is generally positive, it can also blur and distort judgment, resulting in mistaken decisions and behaviors to conceal and deceive so as to prevent negative JCAHO ratings.

Analysis of the details of the professional context is, thus, germane to any management mistakes reduction effort.

Ethical dimensions

Our matrix can also be helpful in limning the ethical dimension of healthcare organizations (Table 2.4).

Nearly every healthcare organization today attends to issues of ethics. At the formal corporate level, for example, codes of ethics, ethics committees, ethics hot lines and consultations, and the like are rampant. At the formal group level, procedures to ensure ethical behavior are typically in place. At the formal individual level, most healthcare managers have attended at least a few ethics training sessions. These formal ethics structures prominently emphasize values that are to be sustained in the organization. The problem, as I have discussed elsewhere (Worthley 1997), is that while healthcare ethics is certainly about values in theory, in reality it is about *conflicting* values, and that modifier leads to some important informal ethics realities that are relevant to mistake-making in organizations.

Clearly the ethical context in healthcare organizations highlights patient rights and professional integrity. In recent years, however, economic values such as cost-consciousness have emerged with force and these routinely conflict with traditional values stemming from patient care concerns. Because the formal context so often minimizes the conflict reality, it is left to the informal level to work things out. When that informal context is not well attended to, mistakes tend to multiply when decisions and behaviors are based on some important values without recognition of other equally important values. For example, is it not true that patients and providers tend to speak of "quality care" often with merely lip service to economics values? And is it not equally true that insurers and administrators tend to speak of "cost-consciousness" often with seemingly lip service to quality of care values?

The extent to which this reality is recognized and addressed is an important determinant of mistake-making or avoidance. Formal structural efforts, such as training that focuses on conflict situations, can be helpful as part of a mistake-reducing strategy. A recent study is instructive in this regard. Schminke, Ambrose and Noel (1997) distinguish *formalism* from *utilitarianism* in decision-making, formalism stressing process and procedure, utilitarianism stressing outcomes. They present the possibility of structuring management decision-making so that both outcomes (for the individual patient/employee and the organizational

Table 2.4   The ethical context

	Corporate	Group	Individual
Formal ethics structures			
Informal ethics realities			

community) and process are recognized and consciously addressed. Their notion offers fodder to those of us seeking ways to better manage the mistake phenomenon. For example, in healthcare, managerial emphasis on the efficient use of medical professionals can easily lead to a process of medical care in which patients are treated curtly and with little dignity. Attention to procedures and attitudes can facilitate a balance so that mistakes, such as treating patients rudely, might be minimized. Their suggestion also applies to the way managers make important decisions when speed seems to offer a strategic advantage. Short-circuiting an open process, they suggest, is more likely to result in mistakes being made.

A corollary of this values conflict concerns the power that fills the vacuum and the general difficulty of managing power contextually. Formally, healthcare organizations rigorously define and control authority within the enterprise. Informally, however, those with little or no formal authority can wield enormous power. We are all familiar, for example, with the way low-level secretaries can have tremendous influence over daily practice. We may be less explicit in recognizing our own managerial power and its implications for the mistake-making issue. When the context is inattentive to the reality of informal power, mistaken use of that power is more likely.

Social dimensions

The context of mistake-making extends outside our organizations to societal influences. First, there are the general social attitudes and mores that we all bring into the workplace. During times when deception and advantage-taking are considered in the vein of "everybody does it," it is likely that such an attitude will infiltrate management decisions and behavior unless it is filtered out by formal mechanisms. The recent spate of corporate accounting deceptions was undoubtedly affected by this social context. Résumé embellishment, workplace theft, and performance hype may similarly be related. As we have witnessed, mistaken decisions can flourish when this context is unrecognized and unchecked.

Second, activities outside the organization are fairly common today and can become part of the mistake context. Managers often serve on boards of other institutions and are active in local community organizations. They also sometimes have financial interests in organizations that intertwine with their own organizational operations. These realities easily engender conflict of interest scenarios replete with mistake opportunities. Social activities can also present potential mistake situations. Association with, for example, groups that discriminate or otherwise challenge social or legal canons can surely impact the mistake phenomenon. Personal social activities, especially for high-level executives, also form part of the context for analysis of the mistake issue. Moreover, the emphasis on cultural diversity within our healthcare organizations has engendered a multiplicity of attitudes that, in turn, can lead to miscommunication and misinterpretation. Mistake-reduction efforts need to recognize and attend to this reality.

Psychological dimensions

Finally, and very significantly, there is the psychological context of the management mistake phenomenon. Executives in healthcare, no less than in other industries, generally tend to bring a sense of competence and self-assuredness to their position. Naturally, a certain "ego" develops the further we advance at executive levels. In fact, the very qualities that mark us as promising managers – such as decisiveness, leadership skill, and confidence – may well mold a psychological proclivity that impairs mistake-reduction efforts.

This reality was brilliantly probed some years ago by organizational analyst Charles Kelly (1988). He convincingly argued that our predominant systems of management education and training, our most touted management practices, and even our theoretical notions of authority and leadership have combined to facilitate a common management psyche that he labels "the Destructive Achiever" syndrome. In this psychological context, short-term efficiency and personal success dominate management behavior and decision-making, and systems substitute for substance. A self-righteous perspective develops (he calls it "hubris") in which mistaken judgment views any means as justifiable for corporate and personal ends of financial success.

In Kelly's analysis, management status and power tend to spawn a certain psychological dementia that includes a presumption of superiority and, therefore, assumes a right to persuade, manipulate or coerce others in order to achieve acceptance of one's superior judgment. The result is a loss of trust and commitment within the unit and organization. The consequence is an atmosphere in which management mistakes are more likely.

Management consultant Jeredith W. Stifter of Hewitt Associates has suggested a psychological antidote to the Destructive Achiever syndrome: a conscious quest of a bias for "diversity of thought and ideas" at corporate, group, and individual levels within an organization (interview with author, London, 21 October 2000). She recommends practical programs that develop a psychological disposition toward *idea diversity*. This would tend to foster a context in which challenge and revision of initial managerial judgments are rewarded instead of suppressed. The context would then be characterized more by openness than reluctance and fear, with the result that management mistakes would likely be less prevalent.

The psychological dimension is a powerful influence on the mistake-making phenomenon. It, too, warrants focused attention.

Conclusion

The study of the management mistakes issue is enriched by careful appreciation of the overall context in which mistakes are made or avoided. Legal, organizational, financial, political, professional, ethical, social, and psychological dimensions are all aspects worth consideration. This chapter has outlined a framework with which to explore the context.

REFERENCES

Abelson, R., 2003. "Chief of tenet owned hospital is indicted." *The New York Times* June 7: C2

Gunn, J., E. Goldfarb, and J. Showalter, 1998. "Creating a corporate compliance program." *Health Progress* **79**(**3**): 62–63

Kelly, C. M., 1988. *The Destructive Achiever: Power and Ethics in the American Corporation.* Reading, MA: Addison-Wesley

Petry, E., A. Mujica, and D. Vickery, 1998. "Sources and consequences of workplace pressure." *Business and Society Review* **99**(**1**): 25

Schminke, M., M. Ambrose, and T. Noel, 1997. "The effect of ethical frameworks on perceptions of organizational justice."*Academy of Management Journal* **40**(**5**): 1190–2007

Worthley, J. A., 1997. *The Ethics of the Ordinary in Healthcare: Concepts and Cases.* Chicago: Health Administration Press: 111–146

1999. *Organizational Ethics in the Compliance Context.* Chicago: Health Administration Press

3

Identifying, classifying, and disclosing mistakes

Wanda J. Jones

President, New Century Healthcare Institute San Francisco, California

Introduction

This is a sensitive chapter. Besides the human resistance to acknowledging mistakes on even a personal basis, there is a severe career penalty to making a clear-cut mistake in a healthcare organization, then admitting it and trying to remedy it. CEOs and other management staff are highly vulnerable as the functional power (read: negative power) in a healthcare organization lies with the perpetual nest of disgruntled physicians, or with the least sophisticated members of the board. Vulnerable hospitals make for vulnerable executives. Just as a football coach enjoys tenure as long as the team is winning, a CEO has a certain amount of job security as long as the organization is making money. When it is losing money, as is common these days (Mick 1990), the CEO is on suffrage. And – is likely to make more mistakes.

Part of the premise of this book is that managers can learn to make fewer mistakes by becoming more conscious and comfortable with the whole idea of management mistakes as having as much need for improvement as clinical decisions. In medicine, professionalism means peer review; in management, professionalism tends to mean looking infallible. Organizations suffer, however, when problems and mistakes are glossed over. Learning is stifled and poor habits reinforced. This chapter approaches mistakes as a source of learning for the individual, the team, and the organization.

Identifying mistakes

When is a mistake a real mistake and not just an unfortunate choice, a bit of neglect, an unforeseen happening, or just plain stupidity? Why not just move on?

The author wishes to thank Ron Davey, Steven DeMello, James Ensign, and Paul Hofmann for contributions to this chapter.

Management Mistakes in Healthcare, ed. Paul Hofmann and Frankie Perry. Published by Cambridge University Press. © Cambridge University Press 2005.

In whose eyes is a mistake a mistake? Some people believe that almost everything executives do is a mistake, since their reference point is themselves alone, especially their job security or income. We will point a little higher – at mistakes managers admit in their minds that they have made. Then, there are the mistakes that others can perceive have been made, but which managers believe were making the best of a situation in which no problem-free solution can be found.

Executive versions of mistakes

For executives to acknowledge mistakes at all, since their culture encourages them to downplay their responsibility for decisions that turn out badly, they should at least have a fairly clear idea of what a mistake is that would cause them to acknowledge it, analyze it, and act to remedy its bad effects. They certainly will not go through any kind of rigorous process for an unclear or indeterminate mistake.

The lessons of 2002 from the corporate crimes of Enron, WorldCom, and others have brought home to the health sector that squeaky clean is safer than concealment. Not only can executives go to jail, but also the whole enterprise can be wiped out for not just financial mismanagement, but from ethical lapses, as was Arthur Andersen, whose leaders and account executives apparently abetted some serious malfeasance and lost their clients' trust.

Executives of not-for-profit organizations are supposed to be agents of the board for both the business success of the enterprise and for maintaining the trust of the community on which the hospital depends for its support. Rectitude is a rusty word these days, but it *is* rectitude – acting from the basis of principle and character – that separates the value-free bureaucrat from the leader. It is the difference between a run-of-the-mill Air Force officer who goes by the book and Curtis Le May, the general who founded Strategic Air Command, who led by force of character. It would never have occurred to him to avoid responsibility for any of his decisions, error or not. Rectitude is what should characterize the relationship between the management and the board itself; otherwise, both can be complicit in mistakes that hurt the enterprise as a whole.

Are we asking too much for healthcare executives to exemplify the highest standards of rectitude? Maybe, in human terms, but for the benefit of a health system with many areas of fragility and temptation, an expectation of any organization in this sector is that its leadership chooses to act in the best interests of the organization and of its patients in both its private business results and in its public roles in each area of their work life and even in their private lives. So, we are focusing in this chapter not on problems that occur in a healthcare organization but on problems that are created for it by explicit management actions or inactions.

With that as a starting point, this chapter will identify the kinds of decisions and resulting mistakes that executives can make, or lead their boards to make, and the kinds of actions that should subsequently be taken.

What is a "mistake"?

A shorthand definition of a mistake: "A decision that leads to negative consequences, which could have been avoided, made by an individual in a position of responsibility, or by a governing body on the advice of that person, or by any other person in a position to influence the organizations' actions, such as a contracting medical group."

At this point, a CEO may protest that few decisions are made unilaterally – they are widely discussed by the entire executive team, surrounded by policies made by the board, and by regulations made by outside agencies. While true on the face of it, such process steps can be used deliberately to "spread the responsibility," to buffer the CEO from accusations in the event that something does go wrong.

For a true "mistake" to occur, it should be the result of a "decision" that was actually made by an individual or a group. There is no point in attempting to encourage executive accountability and remedies for just the unfolding negative events that arise in any business.

Decisions are like musical notes that punctuate the organizational life, like the staffs on sheet of music, providing a framework and structure – or a background hum that helps to determine which decisions will be brought forth, when, and why. As we will see, however, some decisions are made inadvertently when a person in a position to notice a problem and take action does not perceive it, does not necessarily appreciate its importance, or does not believe that anything can be done.

It is hard to run healthcare organizations even in a growth period with adequate income flows. It is even harder to run them without chronic problems in a volatile market with deeply discounted contracts and declining payments from Medicare and Medicaid. Mistakes are more costly and easier to make. The object of this chapter is to help executives make decisions more consciously. But it is also to persuade them that the acknowledgment and analysis of mistakes is a path toward making fewer of them.

Some people may define mistakes primarily as those that become known by other individuals in a position to impose negative consequences. If this is the only part of the definition that would move an executive to take preventive action, then, by implication, it does not matter how many errors or what kind are made as long as they are not discovered. However, such tightrope walking is not appropriate in any industry, particularly in healthcare. This chapter is for those healthcare professionals who are motivated already to do their best; it is to open up the topic, to make the notion of management mistakes one to be discussed openly – and, by example, to sensitize the management team to the kinds of mistakes to consider.

Streams of decision-making: fathers of mistakes

Table 3.1 shows the main streams of decision-making in a healthcare organization, from which examples will be drawn in the body of the chapter.

Table 3.1 The main streams of decision-making

- Assessing the Market
- Selecting Strategies About the Market
- Establishing and Maintaining Power Relationships
- Leading Program and Resource Development in Relation to the Market
  - New clinical needs
  - New medical science
  - New methods and processes
- Demonstrating Stewardship over Resources
  - The operating budget
  - The capital budget
  - The staffing and recruitment plan
  - The site and facility plan
  - Contracting arrangements
  - The land acquisition plan
- Designing and Overseeing Operating and Functional Processes
  - Patient care
  - Energy
  - Finance and reporting
  - Compliance, both clinical and financial, plus risk management
  - Logistics
  - Workforce management
- Responding to Crises
  - Performing public policy role
- Assuring Organizational Competency
  - Governance
  - Management
  - Medical staff organization
  - Knowledge management and decision-making

Every year, literally thousands of decisions are made along the management line shown in Table 3.1; inevitably, mistakes will be made. Some mistakes are those that anyone could make because they were ill-informed, or had too little help, or had never encountered the situation before. Then there are other mistakes, an action or inaction, that any prudent person would be able to say: "That shouldn't have happened." These latter mistakes mentioned in this chapter as illustrations come from the real world of actual healthcare executives, described as anonymously as possible.

Decisions about strategy

The largest category of mistakes about strategy is probably a generalized failure to appreciate the full force of *context* – the environment in which the decision will be made. The organizational leadership proceeds – with the erroneous assumption that the environment is relatively stable and sufficiently comprehended to make the decision at hand. Environmental factors, however, can trip up what would otherwise appear to be a sound decision: "a healthcare organization like a hospital or a health maintenance organization contends with reimbursement systems, both conventional . . . and innovative; with the epidemiology of the population in the service area; with the demography of the population; with the general economic state of the service area; with employers and the coalitions; with regulators at the federal, state, and local levels; with political groups and consumer groups" (Mick 1990).

On a performance level, strategic errors can be rooted in CEO/COO role separation, wherein the CEO has semi-retired to his "Mr. Outside" role, while overly delegating to his COO, who plays the "Mr. Inside" role. Both of them together should be playing a "Mr. Developer" role, but that role is often under-covered and unattended. Tiny shoots of entrepreneurship may occasionally slip up through the budget process, unnurtured, uncelebrated, and unrewarded. A development role would "force" attention to context.

Although CEOs are paid to make a variety of important decisions, those dealing with strategy are especially critical. Therefore, they are worth learning how to make well, with few mistakes. A sign that the CEO devalues this role is the presence of outside consultants writing strategic plans. It should be the CEO's job to think of the questions, the strategies, and how best to present a plan to the organization.

Batched decisions about resources

The budget is really a record of not only many individual decisions, but also of principles of operation and service, of expectations of clinical performance, and a nearly invisible layer of assumptions about how the near future will play out. An unexamined share of those assumptions will be wrong, such as assuming that cuts in nursing positions, benefits, or salaries will be neutral in effect, or that the organization will bounce back quickly.

Five common budget mistakes are:

- Failing to project far enough in advance to reflect expected changes in revenue from market and insurance conditions, so that the current year's budget is unrealistic.
- Making percentage reductions by department, without taking the time to minimize negative impacts from reductions.
- Making deals with doctors "off budget," then finding money in the budget (by shorting current programs) to cover them.
- Committing to dubious programs because of the amount of investment already made, demonstrating an unwillingness to pull the plug early (Argenti, 1997).
- Failure to align contract terms and expenses by clinical program, to create a "business line" structure that can aid in managing resources according to the actual work of the organization which cannot be done by departments.

The budget process does engage the whole management team – but do the members come to the process in a leadership role, or only as the review body of submittals from the departments?

Clinical programs and the budget are the combined "killing fields" where many mistakes are made by individuals and teams who propose changes based on their experience, perceptions, self-interest, sense of competition with other providers, and power positions. Some of those decisions will be right and some will be wrong. "Right" is in the eye of the beholder/sponsor in these cases, where any rejection is classified as wrong, even if it is based on reality – e.g. there is no more money. The CEO's decision-making mistakes may be the result of favoring some programs over others, permitting too little analysis before funding, knowing too little about the technologies either being maintained or acquired, and failing to question demand projections.

The staffing plan is derived from clinical programs, their supporting systems, and the budget, representing a vast potential for mistakes. Hiring and firing are only part of it. Recruitment strategies can be wildly ineffective and expensive. Retention strategies can be wholly unplanned, or mindless, retaining people who have years in service but are toxic to the work environment. Layoffs can result in the loss of valuable institutional knowledge that compromises such modernization attempts as installing a clinical information system that can simplify and speed patient care processes.

The mind-set in the field is to accept the existing range of licensed health professionals and the limitations they place on their own scope of practice, even when executives know these parameters are designed to protect jobs and keep out competition. Hospital-based physician contracts can institutionalize professional monopolies that are inimical to cost-effective care and patient-value pricing. Is it a mistake in the long run not to consider the workforce as a strategic success/failure factor worthy of the soundest planning?

Coding, pricing, and billing together make up the principal communication between healthcare organizations and the payers that keep them in business. The combination of historically arcane pricing practices, the cancerous growth of cost shifts (losses from government programs shifted to private payers), the sheer necessity of pricing so as to attain needed revenue targets, rather than on the basis of cost or value – all these contribute to an atmosphere in which it is all too easy to shave too close to the ethical line. In fact, at least two for profit healthcare systems have acknowledged abusing coding categories to achieve higher reimbursement rates under Medicare. Are coding errors the consequence of a conscious managerial mistake? Yes, of course they are. From hiring and instructing the CFO, to becoming thoroughly familiar with the charge structure and the coding practices, to insisting on deeply probing audits, a CEO lets it be known if honesty is expected or maximizing an unearned cash flow is.

Organizational and governance structure is in the province of the CEO; the board expects the CEO to make recommendations for changes, to recruit outstanding subordinates, and to move quickly when people are performing inadequately. Frequently, a leader can produce a strong governing situation, only to be followed by an executive who allows weaknesses to creep in, inevitably reflected in the quality of management decisions.

Context of management mistakes: processes and relationships

Streams of decision-making are often taken for granted in terms of their processes, participants, and expected outcomes. When talking about management mistakes, it is not useful to discuss only those discrete, large, visible decisions that represent unique events, or the equivalent of creating new lines of business. Executives should look to the continuing, common decision-making life cycles on which the business runs. On the back of that foundation, then, individual, one-time decisions can be considered.

Many of the examples in this chapter are what may be called "one-time mistakes," as they are discrete, are clearly under the umbrella of the CEO and board, and, moreover, could probably be seen to be mistakes at the beginning as they were at the end.

But a large body of potential mistakes lies in the fundamental relationships among stakeholders which the CEO is supposed to be able to mediate. The board, the medical staff, employees, vendors, contractors, community organizations, health plans, regulators – all are participating in the same volatile industry and all have their own goals, their own points of view about what a healthcare organization is and does, and their own independent strategies.

This section of the chapter was for the purpose of laying down the brick road – management mistakes exist, are important, and deserve a professional level of attention. The next section classifies them and gives specific examples.

Classifying mistakes

Besides being alert to the sources of mistakes, or the processes that give rise to opportunities for making mistakes, the conscientious executive should be aware of the range and classes of *potential mistakes*, as to whether they are overt or not, their scale, and so forth. For each type, there should be a *prevention strategy* and a *dissection and correction* process.

As noted previously, mistakes are "decisions with bad consequences." And they are usually those where it is assumed that there was enough information on which to base a better decision than the one that was, in fact, made.

Three classification schemes will help in talking about how to recognize mistakes: mistakes of values, mistakes of role versus performance, and mistakes of size (major and minor). Table 3.1 also shows the subsets of decision streams.

Mistakes of values: history versus the future

Historical values

Hospitals are usually very stable organizations – they have inordinate staying power because most of their stakeholders want them to stay in business, since there is something in it for each one – the doctors, the patients, the local businesses that support them, the health plans that need hospitals in order to market to the community, and even the volunteer board, whose members gain a psychic and community image benefit. That means that such a stable organization carries with it the values of the people who started it and who subsequently carried it along into the present.

Historical values may be explicit or implied in actions, as when these kinds of things happen:

- A Catholic hospital with a beautiful Catholic mission statement of "serving the community for its physical, mental and spiritual needs" does not have an ER [emergency room], since "it would attract people from the Latino inner city community that the medical staff does not want to support" (actual CEO explanation).

- Specialists pressure the hospital to not add similar specialists to the medical staff so that they are protected against competition, even though it means long waits for patients. The historical value set, probably shared by the board and administration, is that doctors must be placated, even when wrong.
- Elaborate mechanisms are created to obtain physician input into the budget, creating changes in clinical programs, with nothing resembling a well-thought-out way of obtaining patient, family, risk group payer, or community input.
- Old clinical practices are allowed to continue even when new science says they are neither harmless nor produce a positive result, such as when mothers and newborns are separated at birth. Fortunately, pressure from mothers themselves – who *do* comparison-shop among hospitals – has led to a nearly wholesale conversion of hospital OB floors to modern labor-delivery-recovery suites that have been highly successful.
- Holding to the concept that a hospital is a "place" rather than an "organization with a collection of services" that can be delivered in a variety of settings. Such a notion leads to centralizing even outpatient services and medical offices on the core campus, even though the people being served are spreading throughout the service area. (See the new JCAHO guidelines for community health, JCAHO 1994).

It is actually very hard to perceive that the organization is holding onto past values beyond their benefit to the organization or even to the public, yet not to do so can be the seedbed of very serious management mistakes. Equally difficult is creating a set of *future-oriented values* that can pull the organization into the future in a sound way. This goes beyond the "vision statement" so popular in annual management and board retreats.

Future values

Historical values may fall short of being enough to guide the future. Either they represent ideas that are no longer shared, or they overlook new values which are promising to be widespread. Thus the mistake is in not finding and articulating appropriate future values. Three examples will serve to illustrate the idea:

- Believing that *alternative/complementary medicine* is still an aberrant movement, and does not deserve to be brought into the mainstream, as both an adjunct to acute patient care or as a consumer business. Yet millions of people are voting with their feet and paying with their credit cards and cash to acquire such services. As many future customers will come from countries with medical traditions different from Western practice, they represent a market that needs to be both understood and served with those traditions in mind (Purnell and Paulanka 1998).

- Ignoring emerging *medical science and advanced technologies* that will make obsolete the current services and programs of the organization, including transitions that will make some of the medical staff's knowledge base obsolete. "The Information Age is not the future; the Information Age is the present . . . There is an arbitrarily drawn curve labeled the BioIntelligence Age" (Satava 2001).
- Finally, believing that the *medical science revolutions* now well in motion – genetics, proteomics, brain function imaging, brain chemistry modulation in mental health, tissue engineering, robotics, etc. – are "not here yet," so nothing needs to be done. Yet, soon one's own personal genome will be known at birth, reviewed periodically for mutations, and generally be part of the electronic record that resides in the ether – and in the appropriate recording medium for the time.

In effect, one is counting on a longer half-life of technologies that had their origin in the 1960s or earlier, that produce large amounts of income now and that are widely accepted. The thought that they might be made obsolete quickly is so frightening that it is put out of mind right away. In mythical terms, the hospital is a Spanish galleon sailing around the Atlantic, while the bright, new Airbus is flying through the sky. In this part of the twenty-first century, holding onto the twentieth century too long is a continuing, multi-fold, costly compound error, that cannot really be subsumed in something so innocent-sounding as "mistake." It is a definite *failure of knowledge leadership*, and will leave the organization obsolescent, regardless of the modernity of its visible assets.

Being alive to history, the real elements of the present, and being greedy to understand the future should characterize the thinking processes of the executive who is committed to minimizing large-scale mistakes on the part of the organization. Lest this appear to be a superhuman task, it just opens up another common mistake – failure to select and educate a board that can provide the necessary balancing act between the past and the future. A CEO who accepts the board, or even the remainder of the management team in their raw, frontier, or even stable mainstream character, risks being ground between 1970 mind-sets and the needs of the twenty-first century. Is it to be expected that a medical staff or a board can be led to be of one mind, and that mind to be always future-oriented? Certainly not. But how much gap can be permitted and still have the organization move forward promptly as conditions change? Does the CEO have no responsibility, some, or a great deal? What would the answer be if the organization were a biotech start-up?

Ethical mistakes

In common with values mistakes, ethical mistakes, especially those of acts of omission, are not often explicit or recorded or viewable by anyone. But they can be more deadly to the organization and to a manager's eventual career or peace of mind:

- A breach of ethics can arise between two parties, as when the CEO demands that a consultant change a report or recommendations and the consultant does so, thus damaging his work product and his reputation, as well as harming his true client, the healthcare organization. The subject in one case was a recommendation that the board itself be restructured because of rampant conflicts of interest. Because the CEO would not act, the board's behavior eventually led to loss of accreditation of the teaching program, sale of the campus, and forced resignation of all but three board members.
- A CEO allowed a conservative board member to order him to get rid of women executives suspected of protecting gay employees on the staff.

Few ethical mistakes are as dramatic as these, but, subtle or not, they can be as damaging as resource mistakes. Overlooking the moral failings of others is sometimes a charitable act, or even a good business decision, such as working through an addict's attempts at recovery. But can a responsible executive keep silent upon learning that a board member or executive of the medical staff or member of the management team has been guilty of wife or child abuse?

Sometimes the CEO has to "take an inventory," as Twelve Step programs say, of her own character as it is affected by the institution being served, or as it is affecting that institution. While management mistakes are addressed openly in the resource category, it is entirely possible that a blind eye is being turned to certain ethical problems. It is especially difficult to hold up a high standard of ethics when the community may seem to be tolerating fuzzy ethics of politicians, union leaders, publishers, professional athletes, actors, and businessmen. Yet, the cost to healthcare executives for not having a finely honed sense of ethical behavior can be extremely high, leading quickly to the end of an employment contract and a career.

Some mistakes arise from capitulating to political pressure from self-interested parties. There are US laws that restrict the nature of joint ventures (JVs) or financial arrangements between healthcare providers of different types who are in a position to affect each other's market share, billing, or profits. Why would one suppose these bills were necessary? Because healthcare executives got into the habit, especially during the 1980s, of bribing physicians to admit patients to their facilities by creating additional sources of revenue for the doctor, based on sharing ownership of capital investments, such as MRIs. Doctors who participated in these projects were often those in a position to refer patients, so could not be said to be disinterested parties. Medicare frowns on such arrangements. Billions of dollars, literally, were generated by these projects, helping to drive Medicare costs to their present unsustainable levels.

"Political pressure" on the part of physicians is a diplomatic term for what is actually medical blackmail. A high-profile physician says, "Fund my project, or I will take my patients to another hospital." Good administrators tell the physician to do just that, knowing that if a concession is made to one, the hospital's assets will be open to others. Or they will find a project format that is legal in all respects. Bad administrators will rationalize their poor judgment by saying, "Everybody does this – I have to keep the doctors happy, and this is one way to do it. Everyone knows they have had their income reduced by managed care, so it is understandable that they should want to find other sources of revenue."

Occasionally exploring such common practices is a good idea for the management team, whether those practices are like the ones above, or are the kind of blackmailing that every surgical specialist does at some time or another: "If I don't get a new laser lab in this year's budget, I know that St. Joseph's will give it to me." These pressures are dangerous and call for the highest level of wisdom. The team will have to distinguish the truly valuable project from the standpoint of the patient, versus justifying the project only because it makes money for physicians and keeps their loyalty to the institution.

Resource mistakes

Resource mistakes involve priorities – with allocating resources among programs, departments, specialties, facilities, or parts of the workforce. Often, these can flow over into ethics, as when a management team does not develop a creative strategy to cover the cost of providing services to indigent immigrant women who come to the ER for delivery.

Resource allocation mistakes are frequently relatively easy to understand when they are large enough to be visible as extraordinary items in the budget:

- A physician who took the helm of a regional healthcare system designated fifty different clinical programs to be headed by both a physician and registered nurse. Each program's medical director was paid $100,000 per year, although no specific management responsibilities were required for that money.
- A CEO with a background as a clinical department chair exempted that department from budget constraints applied to other specialties, and favored growth of tertiary programs at the expense of secondary and primary care, the inverse of community demand trends.
- Another executive approved an investment in a new "cancer institute" outside of the hospital that contained radiation therapy as its core service, leaving chemotherapy still in the offices of medical oncologists. Neither location is geared up for genetic analysis and proteomics, so the investment in plant and equipment is an investment in 1980s technology, because the management team

did not insist on a market-differentiating gain from the capital sought from the hospital, not even for integrated care of patients.

Executives who come to see the organization's budget as their own private venture capital fund will eventually have a day of reckoning, as resource mistakes are more evident the longer they are allowed to go on without challenge. Protection against these errors comes from the right kind of checks and balances, plus a deeper hiring process that spells out the business disciplines the board expects to be followed.

Mistakes of role and performance

"Role" represents the range of expectations of managers on the part of those who hire them, or who are led by them. Roles are explicit in job descriptions, but implicit in culture, custom, professionalism, and the styles of previous incumbents. Each CEO eventually molds the various roles as they are played out in real life. Daily decisions reflect how the executive accepts or rejects role expectations, as when a CEO who flourishes in the budget process avoids any occasion requiring speeches to the public. The core role can be said to be like the captain of a ship, who must continually make exactly the right combinations of decisions to keep the ship on course and away from the rocks. An executive can make many kinds of mistakes that represent a level of performance that falls short of role expectations.

Acting outside one's role is far from uncommon. There is a hubris among CEOs who see themselves as masters of their ships in a Captain Bligh way; this attitude can lead them to audacious behavior that places their hospitals at risk, as when CEOs purchase physician practices – the same practices that already refer to the hospital, so that no new revenue stream is created. To play this role well, the CEO would have to have true entrepreneurial skills starting with a rigorous, fantasy-free business plan, outside advisors who really know the territory, and a viable exit strategy.

Starting the institution's own health plan was a provider strategy of the 1980s, despite the fact that the hospital executives had no insurance knowledge to build on. Many of them compounded the error by failing to lower hospital prices in order to allow their plan to succeed in the market.

An acculturated role failure common to modern-day CEOs and healthcare managers, as mentioned previously, is not acknowledging that they have *developmental responsibilities* in clinical services (as contrasted with compliance or performance responsibilities). They have an obligation to ensure that:

• The right programs are formed to fit the nature and health problems of the community (these programs won't simply arise from the random affiliations of individual physicians)

- Clinical programs are up to date scientifically
- Staffing is adequate to provide timely care that people accept and that helps them
- The medical staff adheres to the highest standards in healthcare
- The necessary resources are made available.

Roles do evolve, but randomly, not necessarily with deep thought and deliberate planning. Role definitions should come immediately after a mission statement, as a bridge toward specifying goals and strategies. Role misalignment can be a rich source of mistakes, since there is no clarity about *what* one should be doing. For example, a role statement such as "provide healthcare services" offers no guidance except to keep the organization out of the shoe business. But "provide a full continuum of care, including chronic disease identification, diagnosis, care and post-acute management" is broad but directive. And it clarifies the role expectation that CEOs and their management teams have responsibilities in clinical program development.

Keeping old programs too long is a mistake of commission; not generating new programs is a mistake of omission. These two classes are worth discussing more fully, as mistakes of omission are the natural consequence of a corporate culture that believes one cannot be blamed for what one does not do.

Mistakes of commission and omission

A fundamental role for a CEO – and, by extension, the entire group of managers – is to *lead*. Leadership is both by action and by example. On a day-to-day basis, the main expression of a CEO's leadership is how inner leadership ability translates into actual decisions, whether formal or informal. People who report to CEOs come to understand what is expected by witnessing the CEO's performance in both the style and content of decisions.

As noted by Hofmann, decisions can be either of two categories – "acts of commission and "acts of omission"(Hofmann, 2002).

Mistakes of commission

Acts of commission are out front – they are subject to a decision process, they are actions, and leave a trail. Usually, resources are involved. Frequently, the act of commission involves other parties who share the risk of the decision. Examination of five years of board minutes will be illuminating, especially if the question is asked: "How many of our decisions had to be reversed?" or "How many would we make again today?":

- The CEO asks the Board to approve a *merger with another organization* with flimsy justification. It ends in hostility and failure.

- The management team votes to build a *new ambulatory care building* around the professional ambitions of a single breast cancer surgeon, who will occupy only 2,000 square feet of a 30,000 square foot building, for which they have no other confirmed tenants.

Mistakes of commission at least have the property of leaving a trail that will permit examining how the mistakes were made.

Mistakes of omission

In contrast, only the CEO may know mistakes of omission; others may not be involved. The consequences can be long in coming and indirect:

- The CEO watches new communities bloom along a new rapid transit route and does not recommend to the board that any additional services be offered to those groups, leaving an opening for *competing organizations*.
- The CEO learns of possible "creative billing" by the CFO's staff, but does nothing since the questionable billing practice is producing *revenue windfalls*.
- The CEO and CFO ignore how physician members of the board are taking ideas developed by the planning committee and developing them on their own as *competitors* to the very hospital on whose board they sit.
- A huge area of risk is run in retaining *marginally competent individuals* on the medical staff, in nursing, or in management. At the first tier of work, mistakes can be small in scale, so it makes less difference if a few people are marginal. But it makes an enormous difference if one has a medical director who is so despised by the medical staff that physicians begin resigning from the hospital.
- Finally, it is obvious that mistakes of commission – actively deciding to rebuild *on the same site*, even though the population is moving outward, can be compounded by associated acts of omission – *failing to stop a project* after realizing it is a mistake, even when all that has been lost is a few hundred thousand dollars of architectural fees, or failing to even test alternative locations.

Better *decision planning* can help with both of these types of mistakes. Healthcare executives might wish to adopt "the war room" approach to decision design (content) and decision management (process) that is used in other industries (Shaker and Gembicki 1999).

Accepting flawed systems

Just as a CEO cannot be blamed for the state of the board when starting the job, there is no blame attached for the functional systems that are inherited. "Functional systems" include the flow of patients between the diagnostic and therapeutic services and nursing; the administrative system that monitors patient flow, information gathering, and recording and communications; logistics; energy; human resources; and the financial system. Here are some flawed systems that were ignored by their CEO:

- A financial system that could not provide *timely reports to program or department managers*, who received theirs a full sixty days or more after the period being reported.
- A human resource (HR) system that spent a great deal of money on recruitment, but had a miniscule strategy for *retention*.
- An operating system that (addressing patient flow among services) required *moving patients among various levels of care* an average of five times per admission.
- A set of department-level information systems on different platforms, with different operating systems and user interfaces, so that care-givers could not find all the information about a patient in *one place*.
- A materials management system still based on *paper*.
- A capital budgeting system wholly based on historical expenditures and a rigid timetable for equipment replacement, but no provision for *deliberate innovation*.

Given that all of these cannot be changed at once, would a capable CEO allow all of these to continue unchanged for as much as five years? When does the CEO become the *de facto* "owner" of these inherited mistakes?

Accepting the errors of others

Perhaps the management team or CEO did not make a mistake directly. Suppose they were total by-standers. But suppose their silence permitted others to make a mistake that harmed the public:

- The medical staff refuses to *rewrite the by-laws* to discipline its members for "economic compliance problems," by which is meant refusing to comply with length of stay criteria, or restrictive criteria on use of MRIs, or rules for billing as a consultant. The CEO allows this to stand, which leads to JCAHO and Medicare sanctions.
- Hospital-based physicians as a class, though in separate groups, insist on *compensation plans* that not only are unaffordable in an era of managed care contracting, but include such monopolistic provisions as the right to over read any kind of imaging procedure, whether done by the attending physician or another specialist.
- The medical staff insists on seeing business plans for new service or facility projects in which the hospital is partnering with a group of physicians, even

though the medical staff by-laws do not give it authority over the *private business of its members*. The CEO complies.

Meanwhile, outside the organization:

- The criminal justice system in the area has a bias against domestic violence cases to the point that *abusers are seldom prosecuted*. The hospital ER sees the problem first hand, yet contributes nothing to the public debate, nor does the CEO or board.
- The proportion of uninsured increases and is leading politicians to put forth universal coverage plans that have hidden *rate regulation provisions*.
- The community suffers from growing *medical–social problems* that do not clearly fall into any sector's area of responsibility, so the failures end up in the criminal justice system.

So, in many cases, the gap between role and performance is an actual ethical issue, or certainly one of character and courage. The management team should examine its collective conscience as to how they believe they should contribute to the resolution of health and social issues that formally lie outside of the organization itself, then set about arranging to contribute in a way that is time-effective and uses leverage-style input where a small amount of effort goes a long way. This is especially true of leaders of large healthcare systems, that can hardly be said to have insufficient power to get something done, even if the problem is large and historically intractable.

As long as there are unaddressed healthcare problems, the public will maintain a certain degree of anger, which serves as a stimulus to political action to exact certain controls on the industry. Having a CEO tolerate an uninsured service area population of 25 percent is tolerating kegs of dynamite under the lobby; you just don't want to let the situation get worse, and, if possible, you want to remove the risk entirely. Not to act on big issues is to accept them when they are essentially unacceptable. Too many CEOs will disavow such responsibility, and especially deny that *not* acting represents a management mistake.

One has only to look at the careers of the healthcare executives who are held out as exemplars; not one of them restricted her work to her institution only, but took a much broader role in healthcare and in their communities – a true "Mr. Outside" role. This may seem far from the common management mistakes discussed above, but this "meta-expectation" is a key ingredient in management success or failure. By performing well in this leadership role, the CEO gains *functional power* that can be used to good effect within the organization.

Acts of commission and omission are both large classes of mistakes and quite subtle. Everyone is not only in an explicit job, but is one fraction of an entire industry, one that cannot be said to be in universal repute or there would be no need for this book – or for such micro regulation.

Major and minor mistakes

A "major mistake" can be thought of as one that is big enough that many people know about it, has large consequences, affects a long period of the organization's operation, and/or reduces its opportunities significantly. A "minor mistake" is the opposite; few people know, it has few consequences, and has only short-term effects. However, patterns of minor mistakes can result in the same outcome as a single major mistake, as when there is a culture of sexual harassment.

Major mistakes

The following are typical:

- A CEO-led merger of two university teaching hospitals without a commensurate merger of their respective medical schools, leading to *early break-up.*
- A hospital set up a joint venture on New Age medicine with a noted author and speaker, in which considerable capital expenditure was involved in order to attract a certain group of people from the community, only to find the center *could not support itself.* The target market had plenty of sources near their homes so there was no need to visit the hospital campus for these optional services.
- Assuming that Medicare would continue to pay well enough that "straight-line demand forecasts" could be made into the indefinite future and that *capital plans* could be made based on those forecasts, even when Medicare had demonstrated regularly since 1966 its propensity for small and large disruptions in its payment stream and regularly even predicted reductions in its future payments.
- Replacing a total hospital on the original, cramped site, so that it was inefficient in design, cost too much, and had no space for future renewal or growth. There was no room for *additional revenue-generating programs* to help defray the enormous capital costs.

Major mistakes can and are often passed off as "The market changed;" "The doctors did not cooperate;" "The board wouldn't hear of doing anything else;" "We never had a lot of interest in this;" "The government made me do it." All such statements should be replaced with: "We made a mistake."

The general problem with major mistakes is that they tend to be system-wide, so they are hard to lay at the feet of specific management people. It is easy to say "not my job." But if it is not anyone's job, then the problems are neglected until they ratchet through the system, ultimately touching everyone in some way, even if it is just to absorb more resources or make meaningful development more difficult.

Minor mistakes

While major problems are neglected, the small mistakes flutter by so fast and furiously that it is hard to catch one, single it out and say, "That's a bona fide mistake." Nevertheless, they can become quite important. The following mistakes fall into this category:

- Placing the "monkey on the CEO's back." The CEO accepts a habit of permitting the staff to "delegate upwards" – so everything is brought to the CEO, no matter how minor. A COO brings the CEO a decision on the color of carpet to select for the surgical lounge. (The habit of accepting the monkey is one that a weak CEO permits because it makes the marginal leader feel needed, keeps the staff under tight control, and produces a false sense of security that the CEO actually knows what is going on. It is a major time waster, and prevents management from tackling really large initiatives. The CEO is always "too busy.")

- *Signing contracts too quickly and carelessly* because there are so many of them, even those as important as contracts with architects. A standard AIA contract may not fit the situation, especially if the architect is hired as a "project architect" with both the client and the architect thinking that the project is ready to proceed to schematics, when no fundamentals have been re-examined. It is tantamount to saying – "Go interview the department heads and find out what they want, then draw that."

- Ignoring actions by individual medical staff members that are *wrong* and, in some cases, *criminal*, such as:

  – Tolerating a cardiac surgeon who represents a large block of business and revenue, but happens to be unwilling to participate in clinical guideline development or use, thus diminishing other doctors' cooperation.

  – Permitting the chief of OB-GYN to *block the recruitment of the female OBs* that market research shows that women prefer.

  – Ignoring the anesthesiologist who *refuses to take calls* from the ER.

  – *Automatically renewing contracts* with hospital-based physicians that contain clauses that guarantee those individuals income not based on their own work, essentially charging patients again for the same service already provided by an attending physician.

  – allowing surgeons to *refuse to order post-acute services* for their sick, elderly patients (case management, home healthcare, and hospice) because "I don't believe in it."

These mistakes, (all real examples), however acceptable to the medical staff culture of the moment, drag down the integrity of the institution and make it vulnerable to JCAHO problems, lawsuits, local scandal, loss of contracts, and board sanctions of the leadership that permitted them to occur. While the CEO thought that avoiding conflict was the first priority, failure to act became the larger mistake. CEOs will say: "I have to choose the number of fights I can take on at any one time." Let's hope they choose wisely.

Strategic and tactical mistakes

In discussing the general category of major/minor mistakes, a number of strategic and tactical mistakes have been mentioned. But it is worth detailing some common strategic mistakes on the part of healthcare executives, followed by similar tactical mistakes.

Theoretically, healthcare executives should be adept at strategy and tactics, since these are the ideas that fuel the operating and capital budgets, and since the concepts of long-range planning and service area planning have been around a long time. In practice, however, strategy is a word that can be denatured to the point that it can refer to replacing equipment to fit the "strategy" of achieving technical excellence. Tactics – the short-term steps to implement a strategy – should be planned to achieve goal success, but may be annual initiatives, where there is no continuity of effort over the years.

Unfortunately, the length of time that these concepts have been employed has not necessarily made healthcare executives adept in employing them. "Strategic plans" are often just goal-setting exercises with department heads, rather than more fundamental changes in direction developed and explained by the CEO based upon an analysis of what it will take to *succeed in the future*.

Strategic mistakes

Strategic mistakes are about fundamentals of organizational success, have lasting implications, and are often not easily undone. Looking back on dozens of what now appear to be serious strategic mistakes, a common denominator emerges of a "compound fault" – the combination of not looking far enough ahead about potential consequences and having a naïve devotion to a planning process that is insufficient protection against the kind of decision that shows up too seldom for the participants to become adept or wise.

Because such large decisions are usually considered the province of the board, the opportunity for management mistakes lies in not preparing the board, not making sound recommendations in small slices, and not having evaluated options so carefully that a cogent argument can be raised against unwise acts. If the board contains a member with particular expertise in real estate, both the remainder of the board and the executive team will tend to defer to that board member, illustrating another common management mistake – not guiding the board to avoid obvious conflicts of interest.

Here are some actual strategic errors where the origin of the mistake is in the dysfunctional interaction between the board and the executive team:

- Assuming that surplus beds were still an asset and that more beds meant more market share, more doctors, and better contracts, so that as demand declined, the hospital came to operate at *twice the capacity that the market needed*. That misconception then directed the majority of renewal capital into acute facilities when it was now clear that ambulatory care and post-acute services were the growth area.

- A hospital board made an excellent strategic decision in choosing to relocate a rural hospital to an intersection of two freeways around which very rapid population growth was taking place. Their forty-acre site was considered a solid investment in the future. However, a subsequent board sold twenty acres as "not being needed." Their hospital and the medical office buildings have quickly *saturated the new site*.

- A province in Canada neglected to invest in its set of teaching hospitals until their extreme obsolescence drove them to face total replacement of the whole set at once. Then, the government selected a small site located in the elbow of two freeways, which could not accommodate all the hospitals as separate facilities; they did not provide the project director or the chancellor with the authority to make decisions about how to cluster or blend the programs into a *cohesive whole that the site could support*, so the plan remains incomplete more than ten years later.

- A Catholic healthcare system purchased a small, low-occupancy hospital in a neighboring small town, and then closed it, so as to force the medical staff to re-affiliate and to increase occupancy at another hospital the system owned. They did not maintain any services, though the town felt strongly about the ER and keeping the offices of local physicians. Because of this failure to consider the *impact of their decisions on the market*, the town formed a not-for-profit foundation to plan a collection of health services, possibly including a hospital, and used the city council to block a sale of the former hospital property. Eventually, the system agreed to open an urgent care center and maintain medical offices. Trust levels are extremely low.

Tactical mistakes

Organizations frequently make tactical mistakes: the kind that can be remedied eventually, but which can become a pattern of the management team, so the sum total may be extremely serious. These are some examples:

- A healthcare system believes so strongly in "consensus decision-making" that its leadership permits the laboratory department head to refuse to participate in an institution-wide "patient-focused care" initiative slated to proceed from study to implementation, resulting in a return to the former model of department-centric care. The failure to implement patient-focused care in this instance led to devaluing *the concept* at the board, management, and nursing/departmental levels, affecting patient care for some years. At the time, it was not considered a serious decision.

- A hospital with an aggressive CFO, who was known to be fond of "deal-making," found that over a five year period, more than a dozen "deals" had been made with physicians and outside providers that had *never gone through an executive team review*. About three-quarters of the deals eventually had to be undone. The CEO felt the CFO was the most effective member of his team, so permitted him great latitude. Both had to leave.

Tactical errors often have political effects far beyond their financial or legal impact, so they should not be approached lightly. Often, tactical decisions are not even made explicitly, but are tucked away unnoticed in the annual operating budget or capital plan.

Single and compound mistakes

Single mistakes

A single mistake is what most people would like to consider a "true mistake" – something crisp and clear-cut. Either you did it, or you didn't. Either it worked, or it failed. Even apparently single mistakes can turn out to be compound mistakes in disguise, but there are some large single mistakes that happen to be relatively common:

- Forming a joint venture with physicians where there is an artistic legal dance around the limitations imposed by the various conflict of interest prohibitions, only to have to buy out the doctors under duress, at an extortionate price, because the business was not a true working partnership.
- Recruiting an organ transplant surgeon to begin a program, only to find that he quickly re-affiliates with the local university teaching hospital, using his recruitment as a device to help him relocate and gain this teaching/research position.
- Opening an inpatient mental health service at the request of the state without an assured source of revenue, nor a comprehensive outpatient care program.

Sometimes when the single mistake is one made by the CEO, the question is whether it is too costly to admit the mistake, if it is not readily apparent to others. This is where a decision-making discipline that at least involves the management team in systematic decision analysis shows a mature regard for the risks of operating a healthcare organization in which so very many high-stakes decisions are made (Heller, 1998).

Compound mistakes

Mistakes often are part of a whole set of problems. In such a situation, it is obvious that trouble is coming, but there is no error-free choice. It is a matter of accepting risk and the possibility of an adverse outcome. The error is in going ahead with insufficient thought about the decision and too little sensitivity to the potential ramifications:

- *Hiring the wrong executive.* The "wrong person" is one whose experience, personality, and character do not fit the organization and which produces inordinate distress for the organization and the CEO or manager themselves. This falsely appears to be a single decision, but inevitably turns out to be a compound decision, because the individual is retained past the point that the mistake is recognized. If the board has made a poor decision in selecting a CEO, it could still be viewed as a management mistake, since the outgoing CEO has neither provided for a strong successor, nor trained the board in CEO selection. The second part of the compound decision is not correcting the mistake early.
- *Keeping legacy computing systems while adding new systems,* justified solely with the notion that this strategy saves money, even though the result is a system that is never fully modern.
- Engineering a merger by creating *unrealistic expectations* that are the opposite of sound business strategy: "both CEOs retained, no layoffs, no consolidation of clinical services, and/or no closure of either site."
- *Failure to acquire property* along a new rapid transit line before it opened, followed by paying too much for it later, and developing it so late that strong competition had arrived first.

A seasoned executive may say at this point, "We went ahead with the information we had at the time, even though future conditions showed that our decision was not so good." In rebuttal, one can point out that the executive pattern is to "discount the future" – to assume that current conditions will continue into the future, so everything will come out all right. What if that basic assumption is simply not true?

Mistakes of law and money

These are both in two subsets, mistakes due to ignorance or mistakes arising from deliberate intent – a failure of character and ethics. The reason for stating these together is that they are so often intertwined, and can bring out similar flaws in character or management methods.

Mistakes of law

Obviously, the nature of the health system under Medicare is that changes in laws and regulations are frequent, sometimes arcane, and subject to interpretation. Management people in healthcare are typically undereducated in finance, so they rely excessively on their CFO and financial staff, plus their outside accountants and their auditing firms. Maybe that should be enough. But one has only to see how general businesses are not protected enough by those resources to realize that the healthcare CEO is very vulnerable if probing questions are not constantly raised and fully addressed to avoid mistakes.

"Compliance" is a growing field of law in the business sector and has become so in healthcare. The advent of the Health Insurance Portability and Accountability Act (HIPAA) illustrates the fact that new areas of legal risk appear regularly:

- The Medicare program can now call on special regional cadres of the FBI to invade a hospital, as it did the Tenet facility in Redding, California in 2003, using a team of forty agents. What was the hospital doing? There were two problems – allowing a doctor to perform heart surgery on normal patients, and using a loophole for calculating outliers that had the effect of vastly increasing Medicare payments. It is quite easy to get in trouble with Medicare, but, obviously, only one way to do everything right – which is to follow every regulation precisely and tell the total truth in any report or record.

- There are whole sets of laws that apply to hospitals as to any business – civil rights, Sherman anti-trust, criminal or tort laws, and laws pertaining to water, air, transportation, banking – every sector of society. Hospitals and other healthcare institutions have a particular obligation to comply with the category of law associated with the professional performance of its clinical staff, as they are usually co-defendants. The management mistake is to pay no attention to the necessary preventive control systems until after a mistake has been made that results in legal action. If managers were evaluated on their risk management skills wherein the organization experienced no losses from legal problems, this success alone would justify substantial bonus compensation.

- Finally, using the courts to settle a dispute that should have been dealt with internally, such as contracting issues with hospital-based physicians, or union contract disputes, where bad relationships prevented agreement.

An inordinate fear of legal actions can be counter productive, a fear that can lead the organization to having its legal counsel exert excessive power and influence, especially power to discourage action that has the slightest hint of risk. Such a practice can emasculate the roles of both management and the Board, which are supposed to evaluate risk as part of their "prudent person" deliberations.

Mistakes of money

"Money," as a broad category, encompasses the sheer control of cash assets, including disbursements, and also extends to the flow of fungible resources between two or more parties, whether health plans or vendors or employees. Financial transactions represent different degrees of trust, frequently memorialized in contracts, and unfortunately constitute a robust set of opportunities for management mistakes:

- In a joint contract with a medical group, the hospital failed to indicate that the hospital would be raising prices during the contract year. The result *eliminated the incentive pool* for doctors retained by the insurer, thus infuriating the medical group and causing it to drop out of the contract for the next year then to re-affiliate with another hospital, leading to sale of the original hospital to a for-profit firm.
- A penny-wise CEO had a habit of *exploiting contractors, architects, and consultants* to reduce the fees they had earned. It might seem like a good thing to be tight for the organization's sake, but such actions may (a) result in those firms being unwilling to be retained in the future, which means paying again for new firms to learn the institution and (b) produce conditions for a lawsuit. Moreover, the organization could have to do business with second-rate firms.
- Accepting donations with *large strings on them*, even though they may consume land inappropriately, produce an eyesore, or be functionally poor is sometimes very tempting, especially when strong board influence is involved. A hospital has a management building that looks palatial, the result of a donation. Another hospital has an education building two stories in height on the last open footprint on its campus, when it has a more urgent need to replace a 1951 nursing tower of seven stories. A hospital built a maternity pavilion only one story high in a parking lot that necessitated bussing employees to a lot across a freeway at considerable expense.
- Another common mistake is assuming the permanency of commercial insurance as the primary source of revenue for the organization, overlooking the trend toward high *deductible and co-insurance policies* and the rapid rise of health services purchased directly by patients.

One does not need to elaborate further about money mistakes – they are made daily. In fact, they are almost a form of "white noise" that permeates the background of every other decision that healthcare leaders make. Unfortunately, much of the industry as a whole is carrying on obsolescent accounting, pricing, billing, and reporting practices. (It took Medicare to bring in accrual accounting to hospitals in its original round of regulations in 1996.) The industry's collective mistake is in discounting the public's angst over hospital prices.

How are mistakes discovered or identified?

When an executive discovers a professional mistake, the next step is often to disclose it to someone else, sometimes prematurely and without due consideration of the consequences. If the executive tells anyone in the hospital environment, the word can flood out from the administrator's office down to the cafeteria and out to the street faster than this person can walk to the parking garage. If the CEO tells anyone on the board, it may be viewed as tantamount to requiring them to take action. If the disclosure is made to subordinates, they may lose respect and become the source of leaks. Nevertheless, not to acknowledge the mistake out loud is to compound it by concealment. How does one act prudently and positively?

In order of preference, there are three main ways that mistakes are brought to light.

Excellent

- Systematic use of *reporting systems and measures* covering both clinical care and functional systems as well as all areas of planned change, such as workforce development and facilities.
- Regular review of prior decisions, based on *evaluation steps* built into projects or based on a regular schedule of internal planning by program and system. The idea is to catch mistakes while the consequences are still small.
- *CEO's own direct observation.* The CEO notices that results are not being achieved according to a business plan for a distinct project, so either the plan was wrong, conditions changed, or management did not perform. (Why should the CEO take responsibility for bringing the mistake to light? Because the CEO has the most experience and job scope and therefore the best ability to perceive that a mistake has occurred.)
- Another manager, or a physician, or a member of the hospital staff bringing the problem to the CEO's notice *privately*. "We have an impaired physician in the ER and the Director of the ER will not suspend him."
- A routine practice of *benchmarking* against best performance by similar organizations, plus literature scans, in both healthcare and in general publications.
- Matters being raised in the regular management team meeting by team members who do not fear misunderstanding or the blame game. (Why place this so far down the list? Because immaturity, fear, lack of experience and lack of true accountability make this method more unreliable.)
- The *board asking questions* that bring a mistake to light. "Why are we pretending that our pricing structure means something, when, according to your last financial report, we discount charges to 95 percent of our patients?" (Mistake: commission, large, compound, financial, legal, etc.)

Standard

- The health system to which the hospital belongs identifies a problem with a decision made in the local facility, or mistakes common to most member institutions, such as following *discriminatory hiring practices*.

- Mistakes are brought to light by a *regular review process*. These include internal audits, external audits, JCAHO surveys, certification reviews of specific programs or processes, and so forth.
- *External consultants or advisors* raise questions during small-scale renewal projects, large-scale systems projects, new clinical program planning, or major site and facility planning.
- Ideas presented at *professional meetings*, through journals, or by conversation with colleagues suggest looking into specific matters to assure that mistakes have not, in fact, been made.

Substandard

- *Insurers, risk managers, and attorneys* bring the problem to the CEO's attention.
- *Physicians* raise issues individually or through their section meetings, or in contract negotiations.
- *Patients* sue their doctors and the hospital.
- The *Medicare program* opens previously closed years and contests cost reports or billing practices.
- The state *attorney general* states that a merger was itself in error or the process used was in error.
- *Contracting parties* sue or cancel contracts.

Obviously, the early forms of mistake identification are preferred over the late forms. This is not "extra" work; it *is* management work.

Mistake disclosure

Communication and process

Mistakes brought to the attention of management by a second party are relatively easy to face – someone already knows about them. The mistakes that are much more difficult and subtle are those that only the CEO knows about, or the CEO and one other person. Concealment can be only too easy. Making the mistake known can be extremely costly. The temptation is to think: "I will just get more information so when I take it to the board I will have a recommendation to make." But if that translates into not making the board aware of a problem for several months, then one's position is totally untenable.

The prudent executive communicates mistakes to those who have a need to know, and are part of the solution. The form of communication is critical, as is the timing and who is involved. This "process" work is as important as the content of the message. There is no shortage of dramatic examples of what can go wrong when initial mistakes are compounded by flawed communications and even worse processes.

Board conflict of interest

- *Wrong*:   The CEO contracts with a leading equipment leasing firm, without competitive bidding, and learns that the firm's CFO is the brother of a member of the board. The CEO thinks the firm is sound and decides just to tell the relevant board member of the lease, hoping he will himself refrain from voting if the lease comes up for any board action on later disputes. It does, and the CEO is reluctant to inform the board.
- *Right*:   The CEO notifies the hospital attorney of the conflict who advises the CEO to ask the board to review the lease and decide whether it should go out to bid and gives the board an opportunity to provide "prudent person" oversight, to disclose the potential conflict of interest and to go on record that the affected board member abstained from any action relative to the lease.

Impaired physician

- *Wrong*:   The CEO learns that an alcoholic ER physician thought a patient was drunk and sent him home. The patient died the next morning from an aneurysm. The CEO told a consultant to the hospital that "The old man is back down in the ER today." That was her mistake – no action in the face of flagrant malpractice by an impaired physician.
- *Right*:   The CEO uses her authority as agent of the board to suspend the ER physician immediately. She calls the hospital attorney, her medical director and board chairman to explain what she has done, then calls the family to express condolences and sends a staff person to assist them with their arrangements. She offers such benefits as her advisors recommend, and does not evade the issue of responsibility. This incident was analyzed by the management team as a teaching example.

Poor contract management

- *Wrong*:   A mistake was made in creating a medical foundation that guaranteed doctors an annual salary regardless of productivity and revenue. The problem was exacerbated by management's decision to carry on as though everything were okay so as not to upset the doctors, the Board or the contracting health plans. Then, when losses passed $70 million, the CEO notified the doctors by letter that their contracts were being terminated. This decision was brought to the board's Finance Committee without notice. There was no prior notification provided to the health plans.
- *Right*:   All doctors were given contracts that spelled out performance measures, options, and an exit strategy, with trigger points designed to be early

enough that the hospital could afford a three-month grace period for the doctors and a three-month advance notification of the health plans. A special task force analyzed both direct and indirect consequences of this program. Reports were made bi-monthly.

Obstetrics closure

- *Wrong*:   A decision had been made to close obstetrics in a community hospital even though it meant that members of the Latino and Black communities would have to use the elite hospital across town or the County hospital, which was despised for its substandard care. This decision was forced by economics, but was not communicated to the affected communities, nor was a mutually satisfactory solution developed with participation by the stakeholders.
- *Right*:   The hospital established planning teams with each of the affected communities and found that the preferred solution was the creation of community-based free-standing maternity centers near schools, so the staff could also provide pre-natal care for teens, and serve as a node of health resources in these communities that were otherwise medically abandoned. The hospital found grants to underwrite these centers and to help subsidize the hospital-based care of complex cases.

These brief vignettes illustrate the wisdom that must be used in communicating about mistakes; the process itself can contribute to either a timely solution or further complications. Therefore, process planning is just as important as content planning, though seldom done carefully enough. The core meaning of "effective" communication is establishing and maintaining understanding, trust, and commitment to action among all the project stakeholders. Not to do that is clearly as big a mistake as choosing the wrong tactical solution. Even the right solution is wrong if misunderstood.

Reporting mistakes: Internal

The formal reporting of mistakes requires that an individual or group in authority be informed of both the mistake and recommendations to address it.

"Reporting" means first agreeing that a mistake has been made, having a solution in mind, and then disclosing both the mistake and the proposed solution to the responsible body. We have spent much of this chapter talking about having a mind-set that is willing to acknowledge that *a person actually made* a mistake, not that "mistakes *were* made." This is not a search for blame but a search for the *point in the process* where the mistake originated. Was it in decision design or in execution? Was it in financial management? Was it in the incompetent rollout of an otherwise perfect plan? Was it in the plan itself, or in the choice of solution, the definition of the problem, or even in the future scenario work?

The first communication step is to the person's supervisor or the executive to whom the individual reports. Together, they determine subsequent reporting as to timing, process, method, and responsibility, and further agree on the depth of analysis and explanation required.

Process

Before analyzing an overt mistake, a combination of *decision design* and *decision process* will help establish a solid management culture that is ready to surface and deal with mistakes. A well-structured decision-making process should automatically produce reports that permit a search for mistakes, then actions on those found. From simple narrative reports to tallies by type of error, a systematic process at the beginning creates an orderly process through the point of evaluation.

Of course, when managers carry out such an orderly process, other parties are quite directly affected. The board comes to understand its role in setting policy that affects projects implemented by management; it does not stay in a false role of micro-managing operations because it does not trust the management team to use sound judgment. Eventually, the hospital staff and medical community come to appreciate the professional way that managers do their work, the openness of decisions, and the fairness of the evaluation process. Both the board and management also have a role in encouraging openness about mistakes, including a presentation of solutions when mistakes are reported.

The budget offers an opportunity every year to compare expected operating results with actual. A project that looked good last year may be untenable this year. Every business unit throughout the organization should have a set of performance measures and targets and be given information on a regular basis with which to make certain delegated decisions, such as staffing adjustments against volume of activity. A *feedback loop* should disclose mistakes made in meeting those targets. Such a process is objective, it is accepted, and it will work with the right education and incentives.

The value of an organized decision process and unambiguous evaluation steps is that management places itself in a "glass window" – people can see in and detect mistakes easily. There is little ability to conceal error. Management will be held to a higher standard than in the cases where there is little understanding of what executives do and how they do it. Since all managers are fallible, and *no* management team is perfect, caution should be exercised to assure that this higher standard does not simply increase the pressure on people to the point that mistakes are driven underground or the organization develops a zero tolerance attitude that sacrifices the person identified with the decision.

Disclosing mistakes: External

Disclosing mistakes beyond the maker or her immediate group opens up a great series of unknowns. Some mistakes need disclosure and others do not. Disclosure is a series of actions, not a single one, because anything requiring external disclosure will have more than one kind of stakeholder, each of which will have different value systems and need a specific kind and degree of disclosure.

Absolutely disclose

The first imperative is to disclose any breach of law or regulation that presents a risk to the corporation and for which the board is ultimately responsible. Failure to comply with a Medicare payment rule, necessitating the payback of millions in revenue, would fall in this category. There is only one process: fast, open, precise, and fully discussed at the appropriate level. Depending upon the nature of the mistake, attorneys, auditors, and all levels of management having any responsibility should be informed.

Other absolute disclosure items include: clinical mistakes causing death or great injury; serious mistakes in handling personnel matters, such as sexual misconduct, theft, or fraud that have been concealed, or where new hires have not been vetted adequately. In the same urgent category would be suspected crimes, either personal or financial.

Serious mistakes are particularly unfortunate and some errors could be considered inexcusable and indefensible. However, all such mistakes become scandalous when cover-up or even the appearance of cover-up occur.

Managers may rightly fear causing people to worry about coming to the hospital because of a wrongful act by an individual, or a broader accusation of fraudulent billing. There is no protection in hiding. The CEO should simply say, "This event happened and our board immediately took action by calling in ... We will bring you updates (daily/weekly/monthly) until the matter is resolved."

Executives should be cautious in taking the advice of some attorneys who will want to limit candor lest it stimulate lawsuits or raise the price of a settlement. They will also counsel against recording any non-client/attorney privileged information that could be demanded in court. If the organization has well-qualified board members, the governing body can be helpful in making sure prudence is not over-done to avoid concealment that breaches faith with the public. What should be avoided is gossip about either the problem or what might be done to those involved, or any legal action.

Disclose carefully

This category includes mistakes in pricing, contract terms, property sales, and decisions that have resulted in failed mergers, loss of high revenue-producing physicians, and failed JVs. Such mistakes should be disclosed to the board's finance committee and/or the executive committee, to any business partners involved, to bankers, attorneys, and insurers associated with projects, and to any affected employees. Disclosures may be planned to limit exposure of this sensitive information to competitors, but only with the guidance of the executive committee of the board. Care should be placed about accurate recording of the actual results in the annual financial report and Medicare cost report. Executives should be particularly careful in press communications, as the bias of the general press will be to search for culprits and emphasize any indication of strife.

Another category requiring careful disclosure is one involving mistakes noted by regulators or reviewers, such as the Joint Commission, where the "mistakes" are of administrative or process matters, not substantive clinical matters that could affect future patient decisions to use the institution. An example of a managerial mistake related to clinical matters would be the renewal of a contract for an anesthesia group that had an unacceptable rate of anesthetic complications for two consecutive years, now necessitating termination of the contract. Such a decision must be disclosed to the medical executive committee and the board, along with the actions taken to select a more competent group of anesthesiologists.

Limit disclosure

Mistakes that involve private individuals in sensitive situations where the organization wishes not to compound an earlier mistake (hiring the wrong person/failure to supervise/inadequate protection of patients, staff, or visitors) by breaching the privacy of the victim should have only limited disclosure lest a new bad act be committed. The entire HR area has a collection of privacy protections that must be honored.

Executives should naturally take guidance from legal counsel, but the situation must be fully explained to the appropriate committee of the board – or, if confidentiality is a concern, to the board officers alone. By documenting in a memo to legal counsel all actions taken, including communications with the affected parties, law enforcement and the board, the executive will have fulfilled an obligation to be forthright in such matters without creating additional potential liability for the organization. As stated previously, the appearance of covering-up a problem can be much worse than any monetary damages that might accrue.

When business matters related to specific physicians are the subject of the mistake, special precautions should be taken. It is important not to compromise a physician's reputation among her colleagues or patients. Medical staff by-laws must be followed to the letter in conjunction with the elected officers of the medical staff. On the other hand, protecting physicians should not mean harming the interests of patient/victims.

It is also important to limit disclosure when mistakes are made in the midst of contract negotiations with health plans, lest the mistake derail the negotiations or lead to a poor outcome. However, if the mistake is so much in the institution's favor that failure to correct it with good information can be construed as misrepresenting the organization's true financial situation, then it must be disclosed to the health plan's negotiating team. Depending on the mistake's magnitude, it might be done privately by having the CFO speak to the appropriate health plan representative.

Disclose at time of remedy

Whole groups of mistakes can be disclosed together at the time the management team decides on a remedy that will prevent them from happening again.

An example could be the form and content of contracts with hospital-based physicians. Taken as individual items, the contracts may seem reasonable, and may appear to be common practice. Taken as a whole over time, however, they may appear to be unsustainable financially, unjustified for the amount of work performed, and lacking checks and balances regarding performance standards. The remedy could be a new management or board policy covering common contract provisions that is implemented in the next round of contract negotiations.

The process should allow lead time for the current contracting physician groups to decide if they want to re-bid or consider alternatives. The whole topic must not be raised for general discussion prematurely, before the board has had a chance to debate a new policy with guidance of legal counsel, to avoid unnecessary waves of political unrest within the medical staff. The board must be knowledgeable about all the issues. They should debate this policy in executive session with no affected physicians present, even if they are board members.

This chapter has covered the nature of mistakes, remedies, disclosure and reporting. Throughout, there has been an emphasis on treating mistakes as an *objective situation* to be analyzed and corrected, not as a search for the guilty. An atmosphere of secrecy inevitably results from egregious punishment, just as a culture of mediocrity inevitably results from ignoring or tolerating mistakes that reflect badly on the organization and its leadership. Good people will leave, and poor performers will only get worse. Executive effectiveness is a corporate asset, just as are the clinical staff, and physical plant.

The management team and mistakes

The CEO sets the standards on hiring members of the team. There should be a conversation that goes something like this:

It is a mistake to ignore our expectations about decision-making, which include how we deal with mistakes. We do not conceal mistakes, nor do we allow our board to learn from others that we have made a mistake. Your compensation and promotion are related to your individual job performance, your contribution to the performance of the management team as a whole, and to the organization itself. I consider you an "officer of the corporation" with responsibility for informing me or one of the other executives of anything you see that you believe should be corrected. My expectations for every manager is that they not only make excellent decisions but that they learn from any mistake made by any one of us. We expect that you will become a strong, principled leader as part of our team, one that everyone above and below you in the organization will recognize as a person of faultless integrity.

Such a statement is at least as valuable as the usual mission and vision statements.

REFERENCES

Argenti, P. A., 1997. *The Fast Forward Pocket Reference, The Portable MBA, Quick Tips, Speedy Solutions, Cutting Edge Ideas.* John Wiley: New York: 214

Heller, R., 1998. *Making Decisions, Essential Managers.* DK Publishing: New York: 13

Hofmann, P. B., 2002. "Morally managing executive mistakes," *Frontiers of Health Services Management* **18(3)**: 3–27

Joint Commision on Accreditation of Healthcare Organizations, 1994. *Assessing and Improving Community Health Care Delivery.* JCAHO, Oakbrook Terrace, IL: Joint commission on accreditation of Healthcare organizations

Mick, S., 1990. "Explaining vertical integration in health care: An analysis and synthesis of transaction costs economics and strategic-management theory," in S. S. Mick and Associates, *Innovations in Health Care Delivery: Insights for Organization Theory.* San Francisco: Jossey-Bass: 225

Purnell, L. D., and B. J. Paulanka, 1998. *Transcultural Healthcare, A Culturally Competent Approach*, Philadelphia: F. A. Davis

Satava, R. M., 2001. Introduction, in J. D. Westwood et al. (eds.), *Medicine Meets Virtual Reality.* Washington, DC: IOS Press: vii

Shaker, S. M., and M. P. Gembicki, 1999. *The War Room Guide to Competitive Intelligence.* New York: McGraw Hill

4

What medical errors can tell us about management mistakes

Carol Bayley

Vice President for Ethics and Justice Education, Catholic Healthcare West, San Francisco

Introduction

Since the early 1990s, and particularly since the publication of the Institute of Medicine Report, *To Err is Human: Building a Safer Health System* (Institute of Medicine 1999), the problem of error in medicine and healthcare has received new attention. What had been a silent embarrassment for the healthcare profession – hurting patients who came for care – has been bathed in the light of scrutiny by physicians and others (Leape 1994; Finkelstein *et al.* 1997). These loyal critics have called for recognition of the difference between a culture of "blame and shame" that has often characterized the treatment of error on the part of healthcare professionals and a culture of organizational learning, one that locates the way to reduce error in the systems and structures designed to produce it.

In this chapter, I argue that many of the lessons learned in the field of medical error can be effectively translated into the area of management error. I begin with a brief summary of the work of two systems theorists. I illustrate some important lessons about medical error by means of a short case narrative, including analysis of it in light of a management policy designed to promote a non-punitive environment for error reporting. Contrasting the "blame and shame" approach with a newer understanding of responsibility for error reduction, I suggest that in both medical and management error, *cultural factors* play an enormous role.

Two Theorists

In 2000, British psychologist James Reason published a short article in the *British Medical Journal* outlining two models for thinking about medical error, along with

Management Mistakes in Healthcare, ed. Paul Hofmann and Frankie Perry. Published by Cambridge University Press. © Cambridge University Press 2005.

an analogy that helped his message to find its way into much subsequent thinking on the subject (Reason 2000). Reason distinguishes the "person" approach from the "system" approach to medical error.

The person approach views unsafe acts as springing from factors such as forgetfulness, inattention, negligence, or other moral weakness. Such an approach blames individuals for errors, as they are seen to be agents free to choose safe or unsafe behaviors. This approach divorces the free agent from institutional structures and systems (and conveniently distances those institutions from liability). In this approach, says Reason, we have no way of knowing where the edge is until we fall over it, since we discourage persons from owning up to mistakes.

The system approach, in contrast, recognizes that all errors have two kinds of causes: *active failures* (of those on the front lines, who occasionally get tired, confused, or depart from procedure) and *latent conditions*. Reason argues persuasively that active failures alone account for few errors. Latent conditions, such as badly designed processes, combine with unavoidable human fallibility to cause most errors. A just organizational culture, he suggests, knows where to draw the line between *blameless* and *blameworthy* error (Reason 2000: 769).

To illustrate the sense of the system approach, Reason uses two analogies. One is that active failures are like mosquitoes. One can slap them one by one, but a more effective approach is to drain the swamp. However, the analogy that has somehow stuck in the literature (and even in error-reduction campaigns in certain hospitals) is the "Swiss cheese" model. Reason says that every system has layers of defenses against error, but these defenses have holes, much the way slices of Swiss cheese have holes. Ordinarily (although by chance), the multiple layers of defense guard against the mistake or error resulting from inevitable human weakness. But sometimes, the holes in the defenses align, and the "trajectory of accident opportunity" pierces through, causing a mistake to affect a patient.

This system approach, advocated by Reason and many other theorists writing in the field of medical error, is reflected in a number of ways in healthcare. The Joint Commission for the Accreditation of Hospital Organizations (JCAHO) encourages risk managers and administrators to conduct a "root-cause analysis" after "sentinel events" (i.e. those adverse events that have caused or could have caused serious harm to patients) in order to address the underlying systems that contributed to the event. A more benign version of the system approach (more benign because it does not require harm to a patient to trigger action) is found in every hospital that uses the tools of Continuous Quality Improvement (CQI) to get to the source of unacceptable outcomes, whether those outcomes are measured in wait times in the emergency department or nosocomial infection rates. I explore this point in my chapter in the forthcoming volume *Accountability: Patient Safety and Policy Reform* (Sharpe 2004), which includes papers from the Hastings Center research project of the same name.

In the writing of another systems thinker, Virginia Ashby Sharpe, activities of quality improvement ground implications of systems thinking. Sharpe distinguishes between *retrospective* responsibility, which is focused on outcomes and blames individuals, and *prospective* responsibility, which focuses on goals and process (Sharpe 2000). Sharpe argues that traditional notions of "quality" in healthcare have been seen as a function of individual practitioner competence and integrity. While that may have been adequate in the days before modern hospitals, it no longer fairly represents the way decisions that may affect patient welfare are made. Prospective responsibility for patient safety, then, resides in the collective that comprises not only direct care providers but managers and administrators as well, since their decisions about staffing, equipment, and policies can contribute to or prevent potential errors.

All of this is certainly relevant to medical mistakes. But is there anything to be learned for managers? The purpose of this chapter is not to apply the systems theory to management – many others have done so – but to show that when one looks closely at medical mistakes, one actually sees management responsibility, either upstream or downstream. To illustrate this, here is a hypothetical case of a medical error.

An illustrative case

Let's imagine that Joanne Jones is an academic researcher and statistical analyst at a local university. She is married to an environmental lawyer and they have two small children. Joanne has insulin-dependent diabetes, which she manages with the same rigor and precision that she brings to her university work. She is strict with her diet, careful with her shots, and she exercises regularly.

Her office at work was recently relocated, so the week prior to this incident, Joanne was loading and moving boxes of files. A quick turn in her new office put her knee in painful contact with the corner of one of the boxes and she came home with a bruise that turned a deep blue over the next couple of days. Three days later Joanne experienced some chest pain and shortness of breath. After a call to her primary physician, her husband brought her directly to the emergency room of Holy Toledo Hospital, where she was diagnosed with a pulmonary embolus and admitted. The ER of Holy Toledo was exceptionally busy that night with several victims of a gang fight and their hysterical family members. Joanne did not put up any fuss about being admitted – she still couldn't get a deep breath – and she knew her treatment would be prompt once she got to the medical floor.

The usual treatment of pulmonary embolus is IV heparin. Because the pharmacy was closed when Joanne was admitted, the House Supervisor went to the pharmacy, obtained both the heparin which was ordered plus the insulin she knew would be ordered for Joanne in the morning, just when the pharmacy would be at its busiest. She took both vials to Joanne's room and put them in the medications drawer.

As it turned out, it wasn't just the emergency room that was busy that night. 4 South, where Joanne was admitted, was filled to capacity. One nurse had called in sick very near the beginning of the shift and the Registry was unable to send someone on short notice. The SWAT nurse would be arriving shortly.

James P. was Joanne's nurse that night and when she got to her room, he got her settled and then prepared the heparin that had been ordered. Joanne was agitated and distressed and he knew that the more promptly he got the medication into her, the more quickly she would settle down and rest. As he opened the drawer to prepare the administration, he heard a code (a request for emergency resuscitation) being called overhead, and he made a note that it was in a room on the other end of the same floor. He was aware that hospital policy was that heparin should be double-checked by another nurse, but with short staffing, a full house and a code, he also knew no one would have the time or concentration to really look. His mind was occupied with who could have coded. Was it the old woman at the end of the hall or that really sick young man just a little down from her? He was glad Joanne was not coding and would feel better soon. He administered the initial dose of 5,000 units and left the room.

A little later, James poked his head into Joanne's room and saw that she was sound asleep. Thirty minutes later, he came to take her vital signs and was horrified to find her cold, damp, and completely unresponsive. He checked her blood sugar level – it was 20. His stomach sank as he opened the drawer. The nearly identical vials of heparin and insulin stared back at him. The heparin vial was completely intact and untouched. Not only had James not given the heparin needed to break up Joanne's clot, he had overdosed her with insulin.

During the investigation, the House Supervisor told the risk manager that James "has a history" of this type of problem. She cites a time when he was a new nurse, four years ago and just out of school. Hospital policy indicated that he needed to double-check something with another nurse, which he failed to do. Although the patient was not seriously harmed, the supervisor admitted she should have written him up, but she didn't, having pity on him because he was new and young. The risk manager checked and there was nothing in his personnel file.

The week before this incident, James came to the defense of another nurse who was being roundly scolded by a physician (who happens also to be Joanne's physician) for questioning an order. James didn't really do anything. He just heard yelling in the hall and went and stood by his colleague. The doctor was furious with him, yelling then at both of them. Later in the parking lot, the physician told James, "Do that again, pal, and I'll see you fired." Forty minutes after learning of Joanne's fate, the physician was in the office of the CEO. He insisted that James' employment be terminated on the spot.

Let's further imagine that Holy Toledo hospital has committed to fostering a culture of learning in the way it handles errors made by staff. To that end, the hospital has a (relatively new) policy on internal reporting of adverse events. In addition to the rest of what one would expect in a policy detailing the proper course of action when an adverse event has occurred, there is a 'safe harbor' clause. This provision protects a staff member from discipline if he or she reports the event within forty-eight hours of learning of it. There are, predictably, some exceptions to the "safe harbor" provision. They are:

- If the act or omission leading to the error is the result of criminal activity or is outside the person's job description or license
- If, at the time of the event, the employee was under the influence of alcohol or illegal drugs
- If the action or inaction demonstrates a reckless, willful disregard for the safety of patients, staff, or visitors
- If it is clear that the employee cannot practice in a reliably safe manner after having been provided with education and counseling.

The first two exceptions are relatively objectively determined. The policy also provides for a particular process to be engaged if the third exception is invoked. "Willful" and "reckless" are legal terms; rather than a supervisor alone determining whether behavior counts as reckless or willful disregard for safety, the policy dictates that a member of the legal department help make that determination, along with a member of the human resources (HR) department. It is counter to a culture of learning to judge the blameworthiness of an error by the seriousness of its consequences.

The fourth exception recognizes that in order to protect patients, it sometimes is necessary to re-assign or terminate someone who is, in the true sense of the word, incorrigible. By definition, this means that an employee who makes even a devastating mistake will not have their employment terminated the first time.

Upstream management responsibility

There are a number of management decisions made before the events of this case began that had a profound effect on the course of events, or as Reason would call it, the "trajectory of accident opportunity." Some of these "decisions" are probably better described as *tacit acceptance*. A good example is the acceptance (or active promotion) of a particular style of work collaboration, without a critical assessment of its unanticipated consequences. The culture that encourages workers at Holy Toledo to think ahead and anticipate the needs of other co-workers also allowed the night House Supervisor to procure insulin from the pharmacy without an order. Perhaps ordinarily the system "works" – after all, if James hadn't been worried about his patient, hadn't been distracted by the code, and had double-checked the medication with another nurse, the system that landed the insulin in the drawer might not have resulted in the mistake. But those other circumstances are less controllable. Distraction and worry are human factors, inevitable and unpredictable. In a way, even James' poor judgement about not asking another nurse to cross-check is a human factor. But if the insulin had not been in the drawer, James could not have given it. This is a good example of Reason's "Swiss cheese": here is a process with a hole in it.

Also springing from an ostensibly benevolent motivation was the supervisor's decision made four years earlier to gloss over James' error in not double-checking a medication – precisely the same departure from procedure that has resulted in disaster now. The supervisor has made two management errors here. The first was her notion that "taking pity" on a new nurse means protecting him from the consequences of a departure from policy, rather than taking the opportunity to further educate him by showing him the seriousness of this departure. This attitude seems to misapprehend the nurturing of a new nurse. Experience can be a great teacher, but only if it is critically examined. Encouraging someone to learn from a mistake first entails the (in)action being treated *as* a mistake. Furthermore, no (serious) harm to the patient the first time meant the supervisors did not take the earlier lapse seriously either, sending a twofold message: (1) the only mistakes that are 'real' are the ones you get in trouble for making or the ones that cause harm, and (2) a nurse can follow policies intermittently rather than consistently, without incurring negative attention.

Finally, when the incident report is filled out on this occurrence, there will likely be a question about whether staffing, specifically short staffing, played a role in the error. That judgment, of course, is a matter of standards and availability of labor, and the presenter of our case has not supplied those details, except to note that both in the emergency room (ER) and on the floor, "exceptionally busy" was the order of the day. Management decisions regarding staffing are certainly a factor in the way a hospital deals with periods of such activity. One can say that in a time of nursing shortages, such as the time we are in across the United States today, short staffing may inevitably result in more errors; one may also say that "too few nurses" is a flexible concept, and that work once accomplished by a dozen nurses is now in some places successfully accomplished only by six. But does that mean that if they just work smarter, three nurses, or perhaps eventually 1.5 full-time equivalents (FTEs), could do the job? Obviously not. There is a point at which making do with less endangers patients, and it is clearly a management responsibility to speak out when that point is reached.

Downstream management decisions

Artificially constructed as all cases are, even those based on "true stories," the telling of this case ends before we know the ending of the story. As such, it leaves unresolved some of the questions that management will have to answer. These questions include what to do with James, how to respond to the treating physician, what to tell Joanne's husband (and who should tell him), what overall weaknesses in the system this error reveals and how to remedy them. Let us look at them one by one.

First, we need to analyze whether the "safe harbor" provision of Holy Toledo's event reporting policy applies to James in this case. James was clearly not engaged in criminal activity or practicing out of the scope of his license. He was not under the influence of drugs or alcohol. His (in)activity in not double-checking the medication clearly jeopardized patient safety, but his action was the result of distraction and a lack of confidence that the double-check policy would have its intended effect – he thought people were so busy that they would resent being interrupted and in any case, wouldn't really look at what he was showing them. Distractions, worry, lack of confidence, fear of looking weak, etc. are not the same as reckless indifference to consequences. Neither was James' action willful; if it had been, James would have understood the consequences of his failure to double-check the medication. The case makes it plain that the result of his failure – that he gave insulin rather than heparin – completely horrified him when he discovered what he had done.

It is an interesting thought experiment to imagine, in a hospital that really subscribes to the system approach to error, whether the only mistake to analyze with regard to the "safe harbor" exception is the one that James made in giving the wrong medication. One could argue that the supervisor also made a mistake that jeopardized patient safety in procuring the insulin without an order and putting it in the drawer. It is clear that the "safe harbor" would also apply to her – this was not willful or reckless disregard for safety and there is no reason to think she had ever been told before that this practice was unsafe; indeed, others were probably grateful she thought ahead. Such is the nature of many hospital procedures (and hierarchies) that this act would not even be regarded as a mistake.

It is clear from the "safe harbor" provision of the event reporting policy that Holy Toledo's senior management has decided, at least in principle, that it wishes to foster an environment of learning from mistakes rather than blaming individuals. Such provisions are designed to remove the threat of suspension or termination of employment of an employee who reports an error if reporting is prompt. In itself, this is an expression of a commitment to justice, since according to the systems theory of error, the employee who made the mistake is just the last unfortunate link in a long causal chain leading to the error. Punishing that person is unfair, when she does not bear sole responsibility for the mistake. However, justice aside, protecting reporters of error is also a practical matter. Management knows that when the threat is removed, reports (of both near-misses and harmful errors) will rise and data included in such reports will reveal other mistakes that are waiting to happen. In uncovering these potential errors, management can act to prevent them. In principle, this is an easy concept.

In practice, however, it may be difficult to implement. There may still be a temptation to blame James. That temptation may come from several directions. The reporter of the case notes that Joanne's husband is a lawyer, not an insignificant detail when most hospital managers consider how to handle the aftermath of a medical error. It may be thought that "sacrificing" James, by firing him, may soften the impact of the error on the hospital's reputation and bottom line. Weeding out the alleged "bad seed" may be thought to preserve the hospital's reputation and limit its liability should the family sue. Even if this course of action provides some measure of satisfaction to a patient or family (and it is not clear that it actually does), it also sends a loud message to staff: we are a learning organization as long as nothing serious happens while we are learning. The safest harbor imaginable will not increase reporting to reveal weaknesses in the system if it is unfairly administered and not really "safe." It also clearly communicates that the financial resources of the hospital are more worthy of protection than its human resources.

There may also be a temptation to blame James if the treating physician, whose patient has been harmed, successfully pressures the administration. Many physicians understand and support the need to look at medical mistakes in a systemic way – especially because they themselves can also suffer when they are at the wrong end of the causal chain – but many factors can interfere. In this case, for example, the physician and James had a history that may have still been embarrassing to the physician and firing James will in effect kill two birds with one stone. It will "make someone pay" for the harm that has befallen his patient and it will remove an uncomfortable reminder from the physician's workplace. Management will need to decide again what message it wants to send.

The other disturbing aspect of this case that management will eventually need to address is the aspect of hospital culture that tolerates a nurse being loudly scolded in a hallway by a physician. On the surface, this has nothing to do with the error. But the fact that James had earlier come to witness his colleague's dressing down suggests a deliberate strategy among nurses to help each other cope with a not-infrequent occurrence: lack of respect demonstrated between members of the medical team. A culture characterized by such disrespect will also likely lack the collaboration among all members of the team that a system approach to both error and quality improvement requires. A culture that tolerates a physician's unprofessional behavior and threats to nurses may also discourage management from following its own commitment to a non-punitive event reporting environment.

Another future challenge for management committed to both a culture of learning and a reduction in medical mistakes will be to address the question of *mentoring*. We have already seen how James' lack of confidence that the double-check system would work undermined his patient's safety. Especially when staffing is short and pressures are high, nurses and others need particular help in learning skills to cope with busyness, including agreed-upon procedures for interrupting one another's work – for example, to ask for help or to double-check a medication.

Hospital culture

Like every workplace, a hospital is the locus of a particular set of traditions, rituals, customs, and power relations, – i.e., it lives and breathes a culture. Culture is grown both deliberately, through the decisions managers and employees make, and by accident, by what is allowed to thrive and flourish, what is squelched, and what flows from strong personalities. When top-level managers (those same managers who are responsible for promotion and other forms of positive recognition) clearly communicate that they understand that systems produce mistakes through poor design much more often than individual people produce mistakes out of moral weakness, lack of professionalism, or laziness, the culture of that workplace exhibits certain characteristics. When senior executives walk around the halls periodically and ask "what have you seen this week that could be changed to improve patient safety?" that executive communicates that there is probably something *every* week that could be improved. Normalizing it, expecting it, asking for it, and making it a priority all establish a *culture of safety* from the top down.

The top-down approach can also be effective in establishing a culture that does not contribute to patient safety. Managers who blame before they inquire (whether it's about a patient safety issue or any other issue) are likely to inadvertently build a wall between themselves and workers. That wall will prevent information for how to improve safety from getting through from front-line workers, where the knowledge is gained, to the policy-makers who can help. Top executives who are perceived to favor those with power (perhaps physicians, or donors), at the expense of those who do not, will have a hard time convincing anyone that the workplace is just and that fairness will characterize disciplinary interventions. This will shut down another source of information about safety and quality, among other things.

But it is not just top management that establishes or sustains a culture. Hospitals are full of informal leaders – nurses and physicians who have the respect of their peers, as both clinicians and as human beings. How those leaders participate in safety or quality initiatives will influence others. Another informal element of culture is "how we've always done it." As evidenced in the case above, established practices may or may not contribute to a positive work environment when safety is the issue.

The nurse who put the insulin in the drawer without an order was thinking about what would be convenient for workers in the morning; she wasn't thinking about the effect of having a medication in the drawer that was not expected.

Conclusion

In a sense, if one accepts the systems approach to medical error, then the actual mistake is the bloom of the tree whose root is at least partly in management policies and decisions. Every bloom contains the seed of the next tree. When a medical error occurs, management has proof that something went wrong in the system – a clear opportunity for management to make changes that will prevent future errors, if the system can be analyzed to reveal where the holes in the "Swiss cheese" of processes lined up to let the mistake pass through. A culture of trust and transparency, cultivated by management and respected leadership, will allow an organization to truly learn and grow from mistakes of any kind. Without such a culture, efforts at improvement in quality or safety will be superficial and ineffective.

REFERENCES

Finkelstein, D., A. Wu, N. Holtzman, and M. K. Smith, 1997. "When a physician harms a patient by medical error: ethical, legal and risk management considerations." *Journal of Clinical Ethics* **8(4)**: 330–335

IOM, 1999. *To Err Is Human: Building a Safer Health Sytem*. Washington, DC: Institute of Medicine and National Academy Press

Leape, L. L., 1994. "Error in medicine." JAMA **272**: 1851–1857

Reason, J., 2000. "Human error: models and management." *British Medical Journal* **320**: 768–770

Sharpe, V. A., 2000. "Taking responsibility for medical mistakes," in S. Rubin and L. Zoloth (eds.), *Margin of Error: The Necessity, Inevitability and Ethics of Mistakes in Medicine*. Hagerstown, MD: University Publishing Group: 183–194

Sharpe, 2004. *Accountability: Patient Safety and Policy Reform*. Washington, DC: Georgetown University Press (in Press)

5

Correcting and preventing management mistakes

John A. Russell[1] and Benn Greenspan[2]

[1]Adjunct Faculty Member, The Pennsylvania State University

[2]President and CEO, Sinai Health System, Chicago

The purpose of this chapter is to provide the reader with an effective framework from which to address the inevitability of management mistakes. This approach is based on lessons learned from personal and career examples of management mistakes, and offers recommendations designed to correct, avoid, and minimize the impact of future management mistakes. During their careers, both authors have made management mistakes, observed mistakes, corrected mistakes, and prevented mistakes. Mistakes are unavoidable if managers are being appropriately decisive. The practice of management is not a perfect science but it has developed a body of knowledge for improving performance. Lessons learned from mistakes, coupled with skills learned in the practice of management, hold many opportunities for improved management performance. In what follows, we will in turn comment on the proposition raised at the beginning of each section.

Recommendations for correcting management mistakes

Celebrating and learning from our mistakes

"For every complex problem, there is a solution that is simple, neat, and wrong" (H. L. Mencken). If we are to be effective and aggressive managers we must be prepared to take risks, to make decisions, to make mistakes, and to learn from the experience. This is the essential quality of successful management.

Management Mistakes in Healthcare, ed. Paul Hofmann and Frankie Perry. Published by Cambridge University Press. © Cambridge University Press 2005.

John Russell

During my seven years as a member of the senior management team at the University of Wisconsin Medical Center, we naturally made mistakes and the hospital CEO, Edward Connors, developed a process to celebrate mistakes and learn from them. The process was called "The Monthly Presentation of the SSW Award." "SSW" stands for "Swift, Sure, and Wrong." All department heads and members of the senior management team were eligible to receive this award, which was presented with great fanfare at the monthly department head meeting. The recipient received a trophy and a plaque for winning this award and retained the trophy for one month in his/her office until it could be presented to the next winner the following month. The program demonstrated that busy executives make mistakes and that we all can learn from these mistakes without fear or retribution. Being the recipient of this award many times qualified one as an expert in learning from, and dealing effectively with, mistakes.

Benn Greenspan

Working in a constructive learning environment represents a welcome but rare opportunity. However, it isn't the only environment in which one can learn from mistakes. Even the most hostile management setting offers the possibility to learn from mistakes. In a different, well-known big city institution the recognized management style was often described as "Management by Gladiatorial Combat." Being directed to "go punch a colleague in the nose" was not a unique experience for us. Such direction can be both alarming and frustrating, but it also can provide a great incentive among colleagues to reason and learn together about the collaborative techniques that improve outcomes and avoid further non-constructive direction.

Some environments may be more nurturing than others, but the point is that any organization can provide learning opportunities to the motivated manager.

Hiring the right person to do the job is a challenge

It is always difficult to assess and hire the individual who will best match the needs of an open job, and also match the personality of the organization and the management team. Recruitment times are usually brief and the opportunity to really get to understand candidates is limited: so is the opportunity for the candidates to understand what the organization expects of them. It is an even more difficult decision for any manager to replace an existing staff member who is unable to do well the job that she was hired to do.

John Russell

When I came to Pennsylvania to be the hospital director of The Milton S. Hershey Medical Center Hospital of The Pennsylvania State University, it was a cornfield.

My responsibility was to plan the hospital, monitor the construction, and get it open. We had very high expectations for this new university medical center to become one of the nation's best. A year after we opened, I took my four top people to a weekend retreat to develop a plan for improvement. One of the exercises we conducted was to rate the thirty-six members of our management team and department heads to determine if any changes were necessary. We were to rate each person on a 1, 2, or 3 scale: 1 meant outstanding, 2 meant doing a good job, and 3 meant the individual was not the right person for the job we had in mind. At the end of a very thorough rating session it was determined that twelve of the individuals were ranked 1, twelve 2, and twelve 3. I assumed responsibility for taking the necessary actions to replace the twelve with the help of an excellent outplacement consultant and we did it in a manner that allowed the person to move with dignity, but it was a very difficult experience for everyone. The good news is that we were able to help those who were being replaced to find new jobs elsewhere and the people recruited to replace them turned out to be good choices. The biggest mistake managers consistently make is to recognize that they have the wrong person in a key position and to fail to do something about it.

Benn Greenspan

Sometimes the reasons for a staff member's failure can make the decision to replace even more difficult. When the Federal government decided to encourage the creation of a new form of federally qualified community health center, our institution sponsored one such effort. It was an endeavor critical to our continuing ability to provide community-based primary care. We reassigned a senior individual I had earlier recruited for another role in our organization, giving him the responsibility for creating and federally qualifying the new entity. He brought unique skills and prior success to the effort. He was once again successful in attaining the qualification of the new organization. Nonetheless, when we shifted into operating mode, he encountered significant problems with the medical staff of the new organization. In the end, overcoming the start-up problems had required many difficult and costly changes for the existing clinics. As a result, he was unable to re-gather the respect and cooperation of the diverse members of the community-based medical staff and bring them together as an effective team. We were faced with the need to acknowledge that his success in one phase did not justify his continuation in the job of leading the organization he had created. While we had to acknowledge his achievement, we also had to replace him. Continuing to leave him in untenable circumstance would serve neither the institution nor the manager well. Appropriate recognition, support, and outplacement served only as adjuncts to the real need to openly make clear the reasons for separation.

The responsibility for building an effective team starts with recruitment and hiring, continues through constant evaluation, and sometimes requires vigorous effort to recognize a mistaken placement and act in fairness to remedy the error.

Making sure your actions can stand public scrutiny

Hospitals may well be considered the ultimate market-/community-driven organizations. The vast majority of American hospitals were created in response to local community forces calling for the development of specific local services. More than half of American hospitals are locally chartered as not-for-profit, tax-exempt organizations. (Most of the rest are government sponsored, and only 15% of all hospitals are operated for profit.) In return for the benefits of tax exemption and charitable status, non-profit hospitals have special responsibilities to their founding and local communities. The traditional responsibility to exercise fiduciary concern for the protection of the assets of the organization is generally well recognized. But the business of operating a hospital has gotten more complex in an environment of increasing government funding, dramatically growing regulation, and increasing pressure to be financially strong. As a result, management teams and governing bodies have found themselves confronting complex business issues that don't always readily lend themselves to the traditional analysis and decisions.

John Russell

Hospitals learned many important lessons about public disclosure from the assault on their tax-exempt status in Pennsylvania. It began in the late 1980s when municipalities and school districts throughout Pennsylvania began to challenge the tax-exempt status of hospitals with regard to property taxes in their communities. Literally dozens of communities filed suit against their hospitals, asking that the hospitals be added to the tax rolls of the community for property taxation. Our approach to dealing with these challenges as a state-wide trade association was to put together a SWAT team of professionals and consultants to offer assistance. The team consisted of legal counsel, public relations consultants, financial analysts, and experienced leaders that would move into each community and aid the challenged hospital in developing strategies and action plans to combat the community's pro-taxation initiatives. The Pennsylvania Supreme Court had established five requirements for an organization to meet to qualify for tax exemption:

(1) It must advance a charitable purpose
(2) It must donate or render gratuitously a substantial portion of its services
(3) It must benefit a substantial and indefinite class of persons who are legitimate objects of charity
(4) It must relieve government of some of its burden
(5) It must operate free from private motive.

Although all our efforts were well developed and well received by the hospitals, many lost their battles and our efforts failed. The hospitals' efforts failed because they could not meet the requirements of the five-point test through full public disclosure. Hospitals that were challenged in court by their local community were required to fully disclose most of their operating practices and many turned out to be very embarrassing. Salaries paid to physicians, entertainment expenses, purchasing taxable property and taking it off the tax rolls, unfair competition with local taxable businesses, bonus and incentive plans to members of the management team are some examples, The Hamot Medical Center (HMC) was the first case in the state to be challenged in the courts, and lost in a big way. Judge George Levin concluded that Hamot met only one of the five tests and the hospital was ordered to begin paying property taxes immediately. In concluding his opinion, the judge analyzed Hamot's twenty plus subsidiary corporations and wrote, "Hamot Medical Center's primary function has been inherently changed. HMC's primary purpose is no longer the promotion of health but to produce seed money for other ventures of its parent corporation. The best proof is the parent corporations master plan which includes plans for a restaurant, condominiums, and private homes." To the credit of Hamot's governing board members, they appealed the court's decision and immediately launched a major effort to change their behavior and to remain tax-exempt. The CEO was fired and the new management team created a plan to reestablish the hospital as integral part of the fabric of the community. Hamot ultimately regained its tax-exempt status and became a model for assisting other hospitals struggling with similar challenges.

Benn Greenspan

Following the rules about public disclosure too closely can be the biggest mistake an institution can make. In the mid-1990s years ago, a clinical staff member with regular critical patient contact tested HIV positive after a needle stick involving an infected patient. The staff member in question routinely had patient contact that was then considered to be "high-risk activity." Immediately upon being informed by the staff member of the lab findings, the institution implemented an embargo of "high-risk activities" by the employee. We then contacted the State Department of Public Health and simultaneously initiated a review of all patient records to determine the pool of patients who had "risk" contact with the clinical staff member. After review of the existing protocols of the Centers for Disease Control, the State Department of Public Health, and the local Department of Public Health, it became apparent that none of the relevant agencies required public disclosure, nor patient notification, in the absence of any specific "sterile technique error." This care-giver had made no such error. After considering the then current anxieties about HIV, the potential for community fear and considering the implications for the trust relationship between our institution and the community we serve, if the news became public, we nonetheless decided that full disclosure (while protecting the privacy of the care-giver) was the proper course. We issued a public statement about the circumstances and initiated notification of all patients having involvement with this care-giver. We offered free HIV testing and, if required, free intervention and treatment. With careful crafting of the publicly released message, there was minimal panic, there were no liability actions, and there did not appear to be any damage to our community relationship. No patients were lost, and the institution received a public affairs award for Best Practice Crisis Management.

The underlying point of both cases is straight forward. We all operate with the consent and trust of the public we serve. Most of us receive large sums of public money and we must remember that we serve the public. We must promote disclosure and reflect it in our behavior. This is not simply a tactical guideline. As Hofmann has suggested in chapter 1 of this volume, our professional ethical principles are merely a starting point. Long-term survival is increasingly dependent on maintaining the public's trust and sense of ownership of our endeavor.

Pursuing objectivity in correcting mistakes and changing strategy

John Russell

One of the essential skills of management is *objective decision-making*. As difficult as it may be to clarify issues, values, and competing interests on the front end of a critical decision, it is even more challenging to achieve this when undoing a mistaken decision. The complexity of overcoming those obstacles is more problematical when you are invested in your mistake. One effective technique is to bring independent thinkers into the process. Such expertise is the staple of successful consulting practices, but it can also be nurtured within your organization if you have created an environment of honest dialog and reward for risk-taking. In either case, the success of the effort is entirely dependent on your readiness to abandon your earlier preconceptions. The right consulting firm can be very helpful in assisting any organization to develop a plan or strategy to correct its mistakes. One of our subsidiary corporations, PHICO, a malpractice insurance company, was having many operational and financial difficulties in the mid-1980s after having great success in the preceding ten years. We selected McKinsey to serve as our consultants; they completed a major six-month study of our organization and its operations and presented a plan to help guide the future directions of the company. They pointed out that the company was pursuing a growth strategy at a time when consolidation was required. They presented a number of operational and strategic recommendations that we enthusiastically accepted. The only one who rejected the recommendations was the CEO who was committed to a major expansion strategy. The CEO was replaced and the new management adopted all of the recommendations. Within twelve months the company was back on track and had re-established itself as a reputable company to do business with. The governing board of PHICO knew that something was wrong and we did not think we could fix the problems without help. Consultants can be very helpful in strategic planning, especially when a process is needed to produce the insights and consensus to achieve the best results or in dealing with a crisis created by management mistakes.

Benn Greenspan

Consultants can be an essential resource in making critical decisions, but they are not the only path to reaching "enlightenment." One of the most difficult qualities to attain as a manager is *objectivity*. As managers achieve the tenure and seniority that accords them the ability to influence critical actions for their organization, they also acquire a natural investment in all of the decisions they have previously made and in all of the people they have developed. For more than thirty years, my own institution has pursued a strategy of redeveloping primary care services through multiple channels in our surrounding communities. We undertook the development of those services because as the original residents left the area, and the economic status of the area declined, the communities had lost their community-based physicians. Without those admitting physicians, our acute general hospital lost its sources of patients. Since there was no natural incentive for physicians to come into the community, we felt it necessary to encourage that redevelopment.

Rather than simply attempt to build one large institutional medical group, we chose to maintain multiple channels in order to mirror the normal, organic nature of a traditional medical staff, as well as to provide varied vehicles through which there might emerge competition and flexibility in addressing a variety of medical care settings. Over that thirty-year period, the strategy has provided continuing success in raising the number of community-based physicians and also in allowing us to redevelop hospital services in a busy institutional setting.

The ability to control various elements of the physician cohort has enabled us to respond quickly to opportunities, and grow. It has also become increasingly expensive to maintain the strategy. As a result, in the early 1990s, we sponsored the creation of a federally qualified Community Health Center. Doing so required that we turn over the control of our physician centers to the new, autonomous, community-governed, primary care organization in return for receiving the benefits of higher reimbursement and eligibility for special grant funding. While we successfully proceeded down this path, we continued to maintain a substantial primary care presence in our institutional multi-specialty group practice in order to retain control of some of these strategic resources.

As the cost of delivering primary care relentlessly rose and the standard reimbursement declined, we were forced to confront the conflict between attachment to an existing strategy that had been successful, and the reality of the increasing cost of that strategy. In this case, we chose to pursue an internal process bringing together all of the parties from our own medical group, our acute general hospital, and from the Community Health Center we had founded (and continued to sponsor). Acting in concert, we were able to identify the joint interests in our community and develop an alternative strategy that would continue to develop primary care for the people we all serve. Our system has divested itself of almost all of its costly primary care centers, relinquishing control of these strategic assets in return for commitments to a long-term partnership with the organization we founded. It has resulted in significant restructuring of our management, substantial reduction of duplication in practice management, and an opportunity to rethink our role as a specialty provider in the inner city.

We expect to revise our organizational behavior in ways that will improve the linkage between our specialty physicians and the community-based primary care physicians. We believe that this leads us into entirely different strategic areas that will bring long-term improvement. These changes required that we objectively examine key commitments that we had maintained for decades and be prepared to abandon strategies that had been the core of our survival. Recognizing the critical nature of the situation, and bringing together the diverse parties, enabled us to achieve that objectivity.

Recognizing poor communication as a reason for failure

"What we have here is a failure to communicate."(Don Pearce, Cool Hand Luke, 1967). This is a statement that can drive most executives crazy. Every member of the management team who is involved with launching a program or action that failed will resent it when someone says that the project didn't succeed because of a failure by management to communicate. In general, we recognize the importance of communication to the success of any organization; yet, we commonly assume that when we understand what we want to say, everyone else will also understand it.

John Russell

In the community where I live, a major merger between two medical centers has been aborted after two years of trying to make the merger work. Many of the employees who live in our community say that the merger failed because the corporate cultures of the two organizations were incompatible and because top management never convinced the people who had to make it work that the merger could be mutually beneficial. The senior management teams from both organizations complained that they held many meetings to communicate the goals and purposes of the merger and that they sent out all kinds of written materials to help tell the story. Management of both organizations failed to understand what people meant when they said that communication was poor. Basically, the employees, the department heads, and the physicians who were charged with making the merger happen said they did not *trust* the information that senior management was trying to communicate and frankly, they did not trust their motives.

Benn Greenspan

Even when the issue of trust does not raise its head, there is a natural tendency on the part of any audience to fill in any blank spaces in a complicated message. When listeners interpret, they will unfailingly do so through the filter of their own fears, needs, or prior experience. Any of us who have raised children through adolescence are familiar with the "Oh, did you mean me?" response. This can be a frustrating factor in communicating change to a large organization. Every individual is likely to believe that the changes are relevant to someone else, and surprised to discover that you meant them. Years ago, in another institution, we brought together the professional staff of our operating rooms to discuss changing our scheduling away from block time for the surgeons. All present agreed that the efficiencies would improve access to the ORs, that the change would save the institution money and also allow us to improve staff nurse and anesthesia coverage. Only later did the parade of busy surgeons start appearing in the administrative offices to ask: "You didn't mean me, did you? I always fill my block time."

Clarity of message is a good beginning for important messages, but it is only the beginning. Important communications must be complete and must be transmitted individually to all of the key constituents. Not only does this improve the specificity of the message, it allows you to assess the reaction of the person to whom you are speaking, and it also conveys respect for the constituent in a way that is likely to improve the response.

Recommendations for preventing management mistakes

Pursue learning and perfecting the management process by using case studies to learn about management mistakes

"Those who cannot learn from history are doomed to repeat it"(Santayana 1998). Certainly one of the great lessons of surviving as a manager is learning not to make the same mistake twice. Yet, the question is often how to effectively learn and how to create an environment that *encourages learning* from a history of both successes and inevitable failures. In chapter 1, Hofmann suggests that health administration training programs make critical use of case studies to promote discussion of management mistakes.

John Russell

Health Affairs (2000) published an article entitled "The fall of the house of AHERF: the Allegheny bankruptcy." This outstanding article details precisely the kind of case study Hofmann is envisioning. It chronicles what went wrong in the creation of the Allegheny Health, Education, and Research Foundation, leading to the nation's largest non-profit healthcare failure. The authors trace the history of AHERF, and then outline the actions of top management that contributed to the system's demise. At the center of the saga is AHERF'S management team, especially its CEO and CFO. Many lessons can be learned from this management mess and the article has become a terrific teaching tool not only for graduate students in health administration, but also for management teams, physicians, accountants, the bond market, and governing boards. The article should be studied carefully by the leaders of emerging health systems to prevent them from making similar mistakes. Articles and case studies about various healthcare organization successes and failures are available from journals, newspapers, universities, and many other sources. Graduate schools in business and health administration offer many types of continuing education courses using case studies as models that can be applied when participants return to their organizations.

Benn Greenspan

Learning does not stop at the door to the classroom. Making the best management decisions, preventing avoidable mistakes, and creating a "learning from mistakes environment" requires an organization that values and practices *perpetual learning*.

Maintain the trust proposition by strengthening governance and accountability

Everything about managing healthcare delivery starts and finishes with the *public trust*. While many healthcare managers already feel besieged with regulation, events in the broad American corporate landscape will have far-reaching consequences.

John Russell

Public outrage over scandals at Enron, WorldCom and Global Crossing led Congress to pass the Sarbanes–Oxley Act (2002). This Act, together with the rules implementing the Act's provisions, now holds public companies and their boards to a higher standard of performance. While these new performance requirements have not yet been applied to not-for-profit organizations, including hospitals and health systems, it is likely that these organizations will be under stricter performance in the near future with the Sarbanes–Oxley provisions providing a template for stricter performance standards. This will occur because corporate governance in the not-for-profit industry has, until recently, been spared the scrutiny aimed at publicly traded companies. As a result, the vigor and intensity of review carried on by such not-for-profit boards leaves much to be desired. Hospital and health system boards must look closely at the new rules and decide which to adopt voluntarily.

The New York Stock Exchange (NYSE), The American Stock Exchange and the NASDAQ Stock Exchange have proposed their own set of rules, many of which are more stringent.

Benn Greenspan

The not-for-profit community should implement many of these standards. The point in citing these standards is not to place further administrative burdens on hospitals and health systems but to suggest that strengthening governance and corporate accountability is a critical step in preventing future management mistakes. It is also a profoundly important step in this era of expanding healthcare corporate vigilance from the Inspector General of Health and Human Services and the expanding attention to healthcare corporations by the Justice Department under the Criminal Sentencing Guidelines. Claims of oversight failures at Columbia/HCA, Tenet, and HealthSouth have only added fuel to the flames that previously led the Justice Department to cite healthcare fraud as the number 2 target behind organized crime.

Some of the rules that boards of hospitals and health systems should consider adopting include:

- Requirement for an *independent audit committee,* with no insiders, responsible for directly appointing and overseeing the audit firm
- Prohibition of auditors providing *consulting services* to audit clients
- Requirement that there be a *rotation of audit partners* every five years
- Requirement that auditors report directly to the *audit committee*
- Requirement that CEOs and CFOs *certify financial statements*
- Requirement that executive compensation and incentive pay arrangements be reviewed by a Board Compensation Committee with attention to the *marketplace for such arrangements*
- Prohibition of *loans to officers and directors*
- Appointment of a *Business Integrity Officer* with direct access to the board and a Business Integrity Committee
- Creation of a *retribution-free hot-line* for reporting perceived irregularities of any sort
- Requirement that there be protection for "whistleblowers."

Many other solid recommendations can be cited, and if implemented could prevent some serious future management mistakes from occurring. The fundamental concept that boards and management must keep in mind is that they are operating in the public trust. If that trust is damaged, their organization could lose its reason for existence.

Maintain the trust proposition by adopting a philosophy of evidence-based management

We have proposed that everything about managing healthcare delivery starts and finishes with the public trust. While organizing the governance functions is a key responsibility, it does not relieve us of the responsibility to make *good decisions*. As we all come to understand, especially since the intense public discussion created by the 1999 publication of the Institute of Medicine report, *To Err is Human: Building a Safer Health System (Institute of Medicine*, 1999), better clinical decisions can be a function of process that injects candid review and scientific method into the decision-making process. We have widely adopted the belief that the risks of bad outcomes from clinical mistakes are too great to allow us to continue to accept medical decisions that are based solely on intuition. So must we recognize that the risks of bad outcomes from management mistakes are equally great.

John Russell

Medical mistakes can have an immediate and awful individual impact. On the other hand, while management mistakes may not impact an individual patient, they can have a long-lasting community-scale impact that may be of greater importance. Management mistakes can diminish the effectiveness of the financial or the clinical enterprise. Management mistakes can weaken the ethical standards that keep an organization pointed in the right direction and supported by its community during challenging times. Management mistakes can even trigger the demise of an organization, causing a community to lose its healthcare assets. So, how do we lower the risk of management mistakes? How do we build recognition that, as with accidents of any sort, some mistakes may be unavoidable, but the risk of making mistakes can be lowered if we are willing to examine and analyze the risk factors?

Hofmann suggests in chapter 1 that mistakes may stem from a variety of decisions (or non-decisions); can be defined in numerous structural categories; may be distinguished by their effect on distinctly different constituencies; and may become evident in various ways. But, despite the multitude of permutations possible in looking at management mistakes, all share in common the adverse impact on the organization and the potential damage to the essential trust relationships needed to succeed. In all cases, how the mistakes are acknowledged, how potential damage is minimized, how events are learned from, and how repeats are avoided in the future are the key to improving the organization in the face of inevitable mistakes.

Evidence-based management offers a structured rigor and philosophy of openness and commitment to recognizing that mistakes are inevitable and must be studied without bias to understand the precursor elements that are avoidable.

Benn Greenspan

In chapter 1, the recommendations offered provide a solid framework that expands on the basic qualities that enhance organizational integrity. The recommendations speak first to the necessity of *openness* that we have discussed above. Mistakes are inevitable and leaders need to create a working environment that allows the full disclosure of mistakes in a constructive process. Our professional and affiliated organizations can play a key role in setting standards and offering protocols and practices that define that constructive process. In the end, however, it will remain the quality of the leader that assures the openness and trust that drives the process.

That authenticity of leadership will encourage members of management to step forward with confidence and present their "learning" mistakes for the sake of helping all of the team to improve. That same authenticity is essential in creating the trust of the governing body that promotes candid and constructive discussion among managers, clinicians, and trustees without reticence and fear of retribution. The goal must be to create a setting in which the greatest motivating force is the quest to learn from every decision and to improve constantly and strategically. As the recommendations in chapter 1 point out, there is great responsibility for the CEO here in creating an adequate *structure* and *process* to assure that this happens. There is also great responsibility here for the CEO and the governing body to serve as "role models and mentors" to assure that this happens. Most of all, among all of the value that a CEO can bring to an organization, promoting a culture that nurtures the scientific evidence-based pursuit of improving management decisions through rigorous examination and learning from mistakes may be the greatest.

Develop a management problem-solving methodology

Consistency in the direction of an organization may be the foremost tool for avoiding confusion and helping to promulgate a strong management philosophy. Achieving that consistency is made easier when the decision-making is reliable and based on predictable principles.

John Russell

Successful managers develop a problem-solving process related to the way they make decisions. Using a well-defined process for making decisions helps everyone on the management team understand what they are expected to do before they make and implement management decisions. Applied properly, the decision-making process will prevent some serious management mistakes. My recommendation for the practical administrator is to develop a six-step process. First, and most important, define the problem accurately. The second crucial step is to select and apply the most promising solution. Applying a likely solution is no guarantee that the problem will be solved; it is for this reason the concept of follow-up is built into the problem-solving process. In order to determine whether or not a course of action has been effective, it is necessary to evaluate the results. Follow-up, honestly done, is one of the aspects of the problem-solving approach that contributes substantially to the administrator's sense of humility. The six steps to my recommended problem-solving process are carried in my wallet and can be summarized as follows:

- Define the problem
- Analyze the facts
- Plan two or more alternative courses of action based on this analysis
- Select and apply the most promising alternative
- Evaluate the results
- Modify the action plan as necessary.

Benn Greenspan

For precisely the same reasons, preventing and minimizing mistakes will benefit from applying *open discussion principles* to the strategy development and planning process in an organization, before decisions are made. Allowing daylight to shine on the deliberations that precede important decisions is sometimes viewed as an unnecessary delay. Encouraging debate can be a troublesome prospect for some managers. The benefits that result, however, are well worth the effort. An openly debated decision that is successful allows other members of the team to understand the thinking that led to the success and to better emulate the process in the future. Likewise, an openly discussed decision that fails provides better insight into the options that will need to be pursued to remedy the mistake. While it may be quicker and easier to simply choose a course of action and execute it without the trouble of broader involvement, no one learns anything from that process to help future decision-making improve.

Make reducing medical errors a top priority

Business decisions are not the only arena in which mistakes are possible. The quality of our clinical product is our first responsibility. The very highest clinical ethical principle is to "do no harm." Preventing or reducing medical errors should be every healthcare organization's highest priority.

John Russell

Solid evidence exists to demonstrate that enormous numbers of medical errors (both serious and trivial) are occurring every day in hospitals and health systems because of "system failures." When an accident occurs it is easy to try to blame a physician or a nurse but a thorough investigation will frequently demonstrate that the problem occurred because the institution did not have proper system safeguards in place. It is the job of management to make sure that effective systems are in place. The Institute of Medicine report, *To Err Is Human* demonstrated that more people die in a given year from accidental injury during medical treatment than from motor vehicle accidents (43,458), breast cancer (42,297) or AIDS (16,516).

The report also demonstrated that the national costs (lost income, lost household production, disability, and healthcare costs) of preventable adverse effects (medical errors) are estimated to be between 17 billion and 29 billion dollars-annually of which healthcare costs represent over one half (IOM 1999).

Benn Greenspan

The report has served as a catalyst to the healthcare industry and the nation to finally bring the seriousness of medical errors to everyone's attention and a major effort is now underway to implement the recommendations contained in the report. In creating the healthcare system for the future we need to move toward a system that meets the challenge of efficiently and effectively improving people's health guided by a fundamental commitment to improving the quality of healthcare. Freedom from accidental injury during medical treatment is a critical first step in improving the quality of care in our nation's hospitals. This kind of evolution in quality is possible only in an environment that accepts the possibility of errors and insists on full and frank discussion of those errors and their prevention.

Appreciate timing as a critical factor in management decisions

The old adage: "The right solution at the wrong time is still the wrong solution" applies to most management decisions. Many examples can be given of management successes and failures that happened because the timing of the decision was right or it was wrong. A decision made too late may have no effective outcome. A decision made too soon can be equally futile. Speaking of his run for the Presidency in 1972, Senator George McGovern noted: "Sometimes, when they say you're ahead of your time, it's just a polite way of saying you have a real bad sense of timing"(*Guardian*, London, 14 March 1990).

John Russell

My best example of the impact of good timing occurred at the University of Wisconsin Medical Center in the mid-1960s when a legislative team visiting the hospital got stuck in the basement on an elevator that was installed in 1926 and needed to be replaced. The Governor of Wisconsin was on the elevator and it took thirty minutes for the maintenance crew to get the twenty passengers out. Needless to say, when the hospital budget request was presented to include replacing the elevators the following week we had no trouble getting the Governor's office to approve it. Many mergers have occurred since the mid-1990s because of rapid changes occurring in the healthcare environment that would never have happened without the current reimbursement climate. Harrisburg and Polyclinic hospitals in Pennsylvania have been major community teaching hospitals serving the greater Harrisburg area for nearly one hundred years. They were major competitors caught in a financial squeeze by third-party payers, and they merged to become the new Pinnacle health system. Many attempts have been made in previous years to merge these institutions but they failed; this time they succeeded, because the timing was right.

Benn Greenspan

Some years ago my institution sized up an opportunity to seize substantial market share through the acquisition of a network of well-distributed primary care clinics. These clinics were owned and operated by another institution which was not located in the central locus of the community-based sites, but had acquired them as part of a larger business deal. It was immediately apparent that the sites would be far more productive as a part of our existing network, and would benefit from consolidation within our operations. The patients of the sites would more comfortably view our institutions as being in their community and would likely make more extensive use of our other services. Additionally, physicians in these clinics were already organized as a single employment-based group practice, consistent with our practice model. Finally, the prize in this acquisition was that there were more than 15,000 Health Maintenance Organization (HMO) patients contracted to these sites from a single insurer with whom we had an extensive and productive relationship. The possibilities for expansion, and the ability to count on existing revenue from a reliable source seemed a perfect match for our cash-poor but growing system.

It is a long-established belief that in most businesses there are only three important keys to success – location, location, and location. This acquisition would give us all three. The success of this purchase carried some risk, but recouping the cost of the transaction required only about two years of continuing business at the existing level, and any growth at all would generate significant benefit for years to come. Within months of completing the deal, the HMO membership of the major insurer associated with the clinics plummeted to less than one-third of its former level, as the corporation went through major disruptions and reorganization. Our revenue fell along with the membership. Our plans for growth were aborted and we have had to continually downsize the network to keep up with the diminishing activity. This decision was on its way to being an unmitigatable management mistake! Aggressive action reduced the losses, but the opportunity lost and the investments made but not fulfilled were never regained.

Location may be "the only three important things" in any business, but timing is still everything.

Know your core business and stick to it

Many organizations and individuals get into trouble and make management mistakes when they stray from their core business or mission.

John Russell

The landmark book, *In Search of Excellence*, (Peters and Waterman 1982), demonstrated some of the critical success factors that made some of America's best-run and most successful companies excel. Healthcare is going through a major period of transition and we see many examples of hospitals or the emerging integrated delivery systems launching new businesses where they have no previous experience, without acquiring the necessary expertise needed for success.

Benn Greenspan

Major mistakes are being made in taking on at-risk contracts for defined populations such as the Medicaid population with no previous experience in managing the health of a defined population. Many would argue that this is part of the core business of the new integrated healthcare delivery systems, but many other examples of strange new business activity can be cited such as: acquiring a medical gases company; starting a new Health Maintenance Organization; investing in real estate; launching new life care community ventures; buying marinas and condominiums; purchasing physician practices; running retail pharmacies; the list can go on with many other current examples. The healthcare leaders of tomorrow would do well to keep a copy of the principles outlined *In Search of Excellence* as a reference for every healthcare management team.

Combine sound management and social vision

With every passing day, healthcare organizations are pushed harder and harder to act in a business-like fashion. We, in management, must attend to profit margins with a rigor that was uncommon in healthcare even in the 1980s. Yet, there is still something special about the healthcare enterprise. We function in a world of singular experiences for our patients/customers. We are reminded that we have a higher ethical standard to which we must aspire. We attend to the needs of people at the first moment of life, the last moment of life, and the critical moments in between. If we are intent on doing our best, even if we believe we are unique, we must look to every possible example for direction and inspiration.

John Russell

In his book, *Aiming Higher*(1996), David Bollier writes about twenty-five very successful companies in America that have prospered by combining sound management and social vision. Some of the companies have blended product innovation with social concern; some have thrived and helped to revitalize the inner city; some have concentrated on unleashing the best in their employees; and others have been models of good corporate citizenship. The companies highlighted range from Ben and Jerry's ice cream company in Vermont to General Electric. The author highlights a bank, a pharmaceutical company, Starbucks coffee, and a little bus company. This remarkable book makes a compelling argument for any business organization to care about the society that we live in and to have a mission of not only excelling at the core business that makes the company succeed financially but in having a commitment to make our society a better place to live. I would also argue that this makes the organization a better place in which to work, and helps management and the entire workforce to be better in everything they do.

Benn Greenspan

Most of us who are healthcare managers have at some time found ourselves hearing (or even saying): "No margin, no mission!" I would propose that we all consider reversing this *non sequitur*. It is possible to provide selected services chosen for the profit margin they generate. It is possible to deliver healthcare services only where patients can be counted on to pay the highest prices possible. We can be "boutiques." We can operate on the edges of the ethical principles that guided the formation of modern healthcare. We can simply be content to serve those who show up in our institutions with a source of payment and to reject those without payment.

There are, however, places where the patients without financial resources need to be served. There are services that need to be available to our communities even if there is no profit margin in providing them. If we want to retain the special nature of healthcare, we cannot turn away from those services and those populations. Management in our field is sometimes said to follow three principles: *Effectiveness*, *Efficiency*, and *Equity*. If we forget the Equity part of the equation, we lose something very valuable that sets us apart from all other organizations. In those circumstances, it may well be impossible to sustain an organization at all without an overriding sense of mission. What then is the purpose of making money if we have lost our mission in the process?

Even in the most challenging environment, healthcare can combine a business-like approach to keeping down costs, to planning appropriately, and to delivering quality. In such circumstances, however, the key to survival may be remembering: "No mission, no margin!"

REFERENCES

Bollier, D., 1996. *Aiming Higher: 25 stories of How Companies Prosper by Combining Sound Management and Social Vison.* Stanford, CA: AMACOM for the Business Enterprise Trust

Health Affairs, 2000. "The fall of the house of AHERF: the Allegheny bankruptcy." *Health Affairs* January–February

Institute of Medicine, 1999. *To Err Is Human: Building a Safer Health System.* Washington, DC: Institute of Medicine and National Academy Press

Peters, T. J and R. H Waterman, 1982. *In Search of Exellence: Lessons from America's Best-Run Companies.* New York: Harper & Row

Santayana, E., 1998. *The Life of Reason,* Amherst, NY: Prometheus Books.

6

A question of accountability

Emily Friedman

Independent health policy and ethics analyst

It is one thing to commit an error, whether intentional or not. It is another thing to be the person on whose watch an error is committed by another party. And it is yet another thing to be willing to be held accountable for either type of mistake, and to accept the consequences. But the truth is that if there is no accountability for managers and organizations, or if there are no consequences that affect them – no matter how devastating the damage done – then there is no reason not to commit errors or even felonies. Accountability and impunity are mutually exclusive.

The psychology of accountability

We learn from a very early age that accountability has a price. If a group of children is playing baseball, and an errant hit goes through the neighbor's window, the children's inherent tendency is to run away so as not to get "caught." Rare is the child who will ring the neighbor's doorbell and say, "I did it." And although most parents, churches, and schools try to teach children that they should "own up" to what they have done, in too many cases that lesson is overwhelmed by experience – that is, once children learn that confessing is not enough, but that consequences also must be faced, their willingness to be held accountable diminishes.

As we grow older, the tension between wishing to be accountable and wanting to run away becomes stronger, largely because the nature of our mistakes is likely to be more serious, and thus the consequences tend to be more severe.

Furthermore, for those who become managers and executives, accountability takes on an additional role. The leader is now responsible, not only for her own actions, but also for the actions of those who report to her. The higher a person is placed in an organization, the more people she is accountable for. At the top of the

Management Mistakes in Healthcare, ed. Paul Hofmann and Frankie Perry. Published by Cambridge University Press. © Cambridge University Press 2005.

organization, no matter where the error occurred or who committed it, the buck stops at the door of the chief executive officer (CEO) and the board of trustees. This is known when people take on these jobs, but even as they say they accept the responsibility, there is a child within each of them who wants to run away from a newly broken window.

Healthcare's high stakes

All of this is compounded in the arena of healthcare, for two reasons. First, most people who receive care from the healthcare system are not patients voluntarily; they have been driven to the system by illness, injury, or fear of illness. They have no choice; they have neither the knowledge nor the technology to heal themselves. Furthermore, as has been discussed widely in the literature of healthcare quality, they usually have little idea of the fitness of the provider to whom they have turned to provide the services needed. Therefore, no matter how much the language of business has invaded healthcare (patients as "consumers," services as "revenue centers"), the relationship between patient and provider is not voluntary on the part of the patient; nor is it an equal relationship. A patient may conduct as much research as he or she wishes on a condition or a surgical procedure or a medication, but that research does not tell the patient if the physician is competent, the medication properly prepared, or the provider organization honest.

The second reason that accountability in healthcare is a special case is tied to the first: precisely because people must trust their lives to the system, they are highly intolerant of errors and misbehavior on the part of providers. When Kansas City (MO) pharmacist Robert Courtney was sentenced in 2002 for diluting cancer drugs that were then given to unknowing patients, the judge told him, "Your crimes are a shock to the civilized conscience. They are beyond understanding" (Stafford 2002). Courtney was sentenced to thirty years in prison.

The combination of patient innocence about much of healthcare, and patient and public rage when healthcare fails, makes for a potent environment in which management mistakes can, and do, happen.

The "no-fault society"

Yet another layer in the complex structure of accountability is the reality of how error and malfeasance are dealt with in the larger society. Any healthcare system is the product of the society that created and supports it; and because it is an intensely human enterprise, the system is likely to mirror that society in many, if not all, respects. The society's attitude toward accountability will inevitably influence healthcare deeply.

Unfortunately, American society, at least, is rapidly evolving into a sort of "no-fault" paradise. Mistakes, misjudgments, even outright felonious behavior are discovered and heavily publicized – and there are few or no consequences for the perpetrators. The saga of the collapse of Enron Corporation, an energy trading firm that engaged in wholesale fraud that cost investors billions and evaporated the pensions of tens of thousands of employees, is well known and is now cited as a watershed in corporate misbehavior. The problem is that with the exception of the high-profile arrest of one executive, nothing happened to any of the now-bankrupt firm's other leaders until more than two years after the firm filed for bankruptcy in December 2001 (*Houston Chronicle* 2004). Indeed, as former employees faced ruin in 2002, a US bankruptcy judge approved $140 million in "retention bonuses" so that Enron could convince 1,700 of its current executives and managers to stay on (Reuters 2002). It was later revealed that, hours before the company declared bankruptcy, $72 million was paid to 286 Enron employees in bonuses; former employees who were not so rewarded have filed four separate lawsuits seeking to recover the money (Associated Press 2003). In January 2004, the one indicted executive and his wife pleaded guilty to a variety of charges and were subsequently sentenced to prison. In February 2004, former Enron CEO, Jeffrey Skilling, was indicted on thirty-five federal counts and on July 8, former CEO, Kenneth Lay, was finally indicted on eleven criminal counts (*Houston Chronicle* 2004). Both were free on bond as of this writing.

Another example, which is actually amusing, is that after telecommunications firm WorldCom was found to have engaged in massive accounting fraud by hiding liabilities and grossly inflating profits, civil litigation between the firm and the US Securities and Exchange Commission (SEC) ensued. The settlement reached included a curious provision: that all WorldCom employees who were involved with accounting, including the new CEO, must take ethics training for at least three years (Barret 2002). It is noteworthy that none of the firm's former executives who participated in the accounting fraud were subject to the same requirement. Several of these same executives were subsequently indicted on federal charges, however (Hill 2004).

Even in the more rough-and-tumble world of professional sports (where, interestingly, more accountability has at least sometimes been demanded of athletes than has been asked of corporate executives), responsibility can be a slippery thing. Pete Rose may still be barred from entry into the Baseball Hall of Fame (at least for the moment), but when in 2003, Chicago Cubs' slugger Sammy Sosa was caught using a bat with cork filling (which is banned in professional baseball), his response was telling.

He accepted his punishment – a minor suspension – but he also started alleging that those who criticized him were unidentified "enemies," that he was singled out because he was Latino, and that, after all, "I didn't kill anybody" (Downey 2003). Given what people do "get away with" in this society, the latter comment does make some sense; but so does the basic philosophical tenet that two wrongs don't make a right.

These are among many high-profile incidents in which people have been caught red-handed, as it were, and have either managed to wriggle out of any immediate significant personal consequences, or else have complained bitterly that they are the victims. And the latter mentality is becoming more and more common. As *Orlando Sentinel* columnist Kathleen Parker has pointed out, an adult must be either profoundly ignorant or severely compromised not to know, at this point in history, that tobacco, overeating, and excessive use of alcohol are deleterious to one's health. She reports that a dozen alcoholics in Scotland are suing liquor companies for failing to warn that alcohol can be dangerous. Her response: "As an American of partly Scottish descent, I think I'm qualified to say: What the heck did you think was wrong with Uncle Rory, you moron?" (Parker 2003).

But the fact is that the attorneys general of many states have been able to convince judges and juries that tobacco firms were aware of the addictive nature of their product and did not inform the smoking public of the risks. This is, at least in my opinion, a valid argument; addictive substances should be so labeled. Whether anyone who takes up smoking these days is entitled to any compensation for ignoring an avalanche of information about the dangers of the habit is much more debatable.

As for alcohol, some see it as addictive, and some see it as voluntary consumption. Sadly, which definition is used often depends on who is involved. As one of humanity's oldest vices – if indeed, one perceives it as a vice – alcohol has long been documented to cause illness, death, compromised judgment, and irresponsible behavior. Yet to this day, people who have made mistakes or committed crimes while inebriated often try to excuse their actions by saying: "I was drunk." But it takes only a positive verdict from one jury, or one judge, to open the door for other lawsuits involving lack of accountability for personal excess. The tobacco cases – both governmental and individual – have reaped a positive-enough harvest that alcohol seems a logical next candidate.

On the other hand, it is possible that the "blame-someone-else" mentality has hit the wall when it comes to the consumption of high-calorie, high-fat food. At least one lawsuit seeking damages from fast-food purveyors for causing obesity was more or less laughed out of court, because, among other reasons, no one has proved that such food is addictive.

A shift in the wind?

So the "no-fault society" may actually have some limits. But, for the most part, the societal environment in which the healthcare executive must navigate is one in which there is little reward for admitting error, and a great deal of reward for concealing it; where the consequences of mistakes or misbehavior can be slight, and the monetary compensation sizeable; and where, if it is possible to blame someone else for our own actions, we will.

At the same time, there are whispers of change. Although Samuel Waksal, former CEO of Imclone (a pharmaceutical firm involved in stock fraud) was the first executive involved in any of the major corporate scandals of the twenty-first century to actually be sentenced to prison, other high-profile miscreants, including the well-known celebrity, Martha Stewart, have met the same fate more recently and several corporations have been fined and otherwise penalized for their actions (Hays 2004). The SEC, which has been extremely lenient with many of these firms, now requires that CEOs personally attest to the correctness of their companies' financial reports.

Perhaps more important is that publicly held firms have suffered a backlash in public confidence. A *Chicago Tribune* poll conducted in 2002 found that 42% of respondents had "very little" or "no" confidence in top corporate executives; 76% believed that top corporate executives "put their own personal interests ahead of the interests of workers and shareholders"; and 66% believed that "compared with 10 to 20 years ago, the ethical standards of major corporation executives have changed for the worse" (Burns 2002).

Lack of public confidence may not lead to indictment or prosecution, but it can most certainly affect stock prices, community support, and the solvency of a firm. That, more than any minor fine, can be a force for change. Indeed, in a three-month period in late 2002, at least 100 US firms hired ethics officers. There is now an Ethics Officer Association, whose members represent half of the *Fortune* 500, the World Bank, and the New York Stock Exchange (NYSE) (Salant 2002).

Whether hiring an ethics officer is for show or for real is, of course, a matter of debate. Which it is depends, in large measure, on that officer's power and the level of support she enjoys from top leadership. There is also the crucial question of whether the ethics effort involves simply attempting to comply with law or regulation, or whether it goes further to attempt to establish an *ethical and accountable organization* with ethical and accountable leadership. In one recent case, a large propriety hospital firm that had been found to have committed extensive fraud against government programs and private insurers hired a compliance expert from the Department of Defense – which has had more than a few scandals of its own – and named him their chief ethics officer. The perception of many observers was that the firm's leadership believed that compliance with the law is the same as ethical integrity, a stance with which many might disagree.

The healthcare environment

Certainly the larger social environment is placing significant obstacles in the path of the accountable healthcare executive seeking to build an accountable organization – and that is on top of the challenges that already exist. And it is evident that not all healthcare executives and organizations are, indeed, seeking to establish accountability.

When two cardiac surgeons at a Redding, California, hospital owned by Tenet Healthcare, a for-profit firm, were accused of performing unnecessary and risky operations on patients, a Tenet spokesman commented that "this is an investigation of doctors, not the hospital or Tenet" (Lee and White 2002). However, another cardiologist practicing at the same hospital alleged that hospital executives "looked the other way 'because [the two surgeons] produce tremendous revenue for the hospital.'" The hospital reportedly generated a net profit of 38%, which is extraordinarily high for any healthcare facility. In August 2003, despite its previous claims that it had nothing to do with the situation, Tenet agreed to pay $54 million in fines to the Federal government and the state of California (Appleby 2003). Tenet, the Redding hospital, and the two surgeons, were also facing some 100 civil lawsuits filed by patients and families (Vrana and White 2003).

Despite its apparent culpability in the Redding matter, Tenet retained its "who, me?" corporate attitude. When some Tenet hospitals were accused of Medicare fraud in 2003, the parent company issued a statement urging the US Department of Justice to file suit against the individual hospitals and not the corporate parent, arguing that the federal government had used "global" criteria as the basis for its complaint, rather than "a statistical analysis for each hospital" (*Kaiser Daily Health Policy Report* 2003).

It would be difficult to find a more blatant example of leadership at the top of a healthcare enterprise seeking to distance itself from the actions of those whom it oversees – especially when those subsidiary entities, and their actions, form the basis for the parent firm's financial performance and its standing in the market. This apparently did not go unnoticed; in January 2004, in the face of declining stock prices, Tenet announced that it was selling twenty-seven of its hospitals, including the one in Redding, which was sold in July (Associated Press 2004).

Another, and equally upsetting, example, is that of HealthSouth, another publicly owned healthcare firm, which is embroiled in several scandals involving accounting and tax fraud and financial irregularities. In response to SEC inquiries about the role of the CEO, Richard Scrushy, his attorneys argued that he had no responsibility for what had happened, because, they said, he was an absentee executive who spent most of his time on his estate in Palm Beach, Florida, and had little involvement with the company. One attorney, Thomas Sjoblom, stated, "It's a mistake to say he was a hands-on manager" (Farrell 2003). The organization certainly does not seem to have had a model chain of command. Michael Vines, a bookkeeper at HealthSouth, had realized that there were gross accounting irregularities at the firm and had attempted to report them within the firm; his allegations were ignored. He then informed the company's outside auditor, which dismissed his concerns. He finally turned to posting his protests on the Internet. In 2003, the former chief financial officer of HealthSouth pleaded guilty to fraud in a criminal case against the firm; the SEC has filed a civil complaint (Mollenkamp 2003). It has since been revealed that HealthSouth classified $2.6 million in payments for janitorial services as "audit-related fees," and the firm's external auditor stated that this was a proper accounting (Reuters 2003). As of August 2003, fourteen HealthSouth executives, including all five of the CFOs the firm has had in its existence, had pleaded guilty to financial crime (Galloro 2003). In November 2003, Scrushy was indicted on eighty-five federal criminal counts (Ackman 2003).

Does it matter?

At this juncture, the question might well be asked: Why should a healthcare executive be accountable for her actions and those of her employees? What good can come of trying to establish an accountable organization in the midst of what appears to be a corporate ethics meltdown, in and out of healthcare?

There are several sound reasons for pursuing these laudable but admittedly challenging goals. The first is that, sooner or later, especially in healthcare, wrongdoing is discovered and penalized. We may gnash our teeth at the ponderously slow process and the escape from justice of some culpable individuals, but in the long term, organizations that commit fraud and other forms of harm suffer penalties, if not in formal proceedings, then at the hands of the public, communities, and investors. And sooner or later, lawsuits by individual members of the public who believe they have been harmed are inevitable.

Second, healthcare organizations depend, to an extraordinary degree, on the good will of their publics and their communities. There is more than one instance of a hospital or clinic or health plan that is found to have violated public trust that is no longer in operation. On a more mundane level, there is always the need for payer contracts, construction permits, easements, philanthropic donations – and patients. Once a healthcare provider or payer is perceived to be untrustworthy, the perception of what it deserves shifts, and it can take generations before that perception changes.

Third, although the argument sometimes sounds hollow, being perceived as "trustworthy" is a market advantage, especially in healthcare. As Jim Berg, director of ethics and business practice for International Paper, has said, "If you have a reputation for ethical behavior, that, in today's marketplace, is a competitive advantage. It engenders not only customer loyalty, but employee loyalty" (Salant 2002).

Fourth, as the above quote indicates, a reputation for integrity is a bonus in an increasingly tight healthcare employment market. An organization that, for example, is known to tolerate sexual harassment and racial discrimination is hardly going to be an appealing employer in a century in which healthcare will be even more dependent on female and minority workers. For graduates of business and health administration schools, working for an organization that is under investigation or indictment is not a very attractive prospect.

Fifth, as is being discussed urgently in healthcare circles, payers and patients alike are pushing for higher quality and reliability in patient care. Accountability is a quality-of-care issue. Healthcare organizations that refuse to admit errors and seek to cover them up, that blame scapegoats, or that look the other way in the face of obvious mistakes are not likely to survive the coming era of accountability for quality of care. In almost every scandal that has erupted, there are implications for patient safety and outcomes of care, whether the problem is using underskilled staff, falsifying medical records, performing unnecessary or dangerous procedures, or sucking money away from patient care into individual or corporate private pockets. As has been discussed, the public will take a dim view indeed of management decisions that provoke such consequences.

Sixth, it is exceedingly rare that a healthcare executive spends his or her entire career in one organization. Even if one is not "caught" by the SEC, the Department of Justice, or the local police, healthcare administration is a somewhat small and exclusive club; what one has done, or not done, will haunt any executive in future job searches. Rare is the board of trustees that will even consider a candidate with a clouded past.

Seventh – even if it seems out of place in times such as these – being true to a moral code allows one to live a happier life and to lead a happier organization. There are intense personal rewards for those who choose the higher road, not the least of which is being highly regarded by one's peers and employees – and being able to sleep at night. As the Beatles sang, money can't buy you love.

Establishing accountable leadership

There are several means by which a healthcare executive can establish accountability for herself and her peers.

First, know who are you hiring and ask questions about ethics. Describing integrity in leadership as "the real bottom line," David Canfield wrote: "Whether building a senior management team or hiring a new college graduate, healthcare executives should make integrity a prerequisite. Ask candidates to describe ethical dilemmas they have faced and how they handled them. Ask references about a candidate's character. And let's not forget the team you already have. Make sure they understand that integrity, not financial success, is Job One" (Canfield 2003).

Second, don't trust to the fates. There must be oversight of executive performance and decision-making, and a means of reporting failure, just in case the executive in question is shy about reporting on herself. This should be a responsibility of the board, but if there is any question about the board's commitment to ethical oversight, the process should be internal to the executive suite.

Third, what happens when there is a problem? Do other executives and employees recoil in fear at the idea of reporting or commenting on or trying to respond to a management mistake? Is there a process in place for limiting harm, investigating what happened, and seeking to prevent such occurrences in the future? Or is there a rush to cover the whole thing up?

Fourth, is there an executive culture that encourages facing consequences, or rewards avoiding them? Extremely important here is the long-time practice of indemnifying trustees, and often executives, against the consequences of their actions. If a leader is guaranteed a handsome income, no matter what she does or what the consequences are, then accountability is zero. Similarly, "platinum parachutes" and glowing recommendations for someone who has failed as a leader and whom the organization is just trying to get rid of hardly encourage a culture of accountability.

It is not enough to say that one is accountable for one's actions; there must be tangible evidence that something is on the line, that one's "skin is in the game." Yet that is not always the case. On one end of the spectrum, there are healthcare executives who have engaged in serious financial mismanagement and fraud – and who walk away with millions of dollars; at the other end are healthcare executives who have tied their future compensation to improvements in the overall health of the communities they serve. Which type of organization – and its leaders – is likely to stand the test of time?

Another aspect of this is that if the organization and its leadership fail to establish both accountability and responsibility for the consequences of their actions and of those whom they oversee, it is highly likely that, in the event of mistake or failure, external entities – including government, attorneys, and/or and the market – will step into the vacuum thus created.

Fifth, it is necessary to have a chain of accountability. In a "no-fault" society, the search for villains can consume a great deal of utterly wasted time. Yet, as in the examples presented earlier, a common response to being found in error is to abjure responsibility and accuse one's subordinates, affiliated organizations, "enemies,' bigots, or the lamp post. Indeed, healthcare organizations and entire systems have become adept at avoiding accountability for any problem that cannot be absolutely laid at their feet. A recent example has been the search for the cause of the current spike in healthcare inflation after a few years of relative calm. One study blamed health plans, most of which have returned to financial health and even record profits; another blamed hospitals; another blamed rising pharmaceutical costs. Each alleged perpetrator immediately accused one of the others, and the healthcare press – and sometimes the public press – was soon inundated with dueling studies. All of the accused have played a role in skyrocketing healthcare costs; but it would be more sensible, and certainly more humane, to focus instead on how those prices could be brought under control instead of trying to deflect attention from oneself so that one can hang onto one's piece of the pie.

When a healthcare executive assumes a leadership position, it is assumed that she is also assuming responsibility for the actions of those under her. The executive is also responsible for the consequences of those actions. Those leaders who prefer to blame individual elements of their organizations, or to claim ignorance (which, as the law states, is no excuse), or to break the chain of accountability, are not fit for command. As James Battles reminds us, healthcare organizations include people who provide direct care and services, whom he refers to as "sharp ends," and people who run the enterprise but do not provide direct care, such as executives, managers, and board members, whom he refers to as "blunt ends." His advice is that "if you hold 'sharp end' individuals accountable for their actions and decisions, you must also make 'blunt end' individuals accountable for their actions and decisions" (Friedman 2001).

Establishing an accountable organization

But accountable leadership is not enough – and, indeed, such leadership will not last long if it is not presiding over an accountable organization. And despite the dizzying complexity of healthcare organizations and their hundreds, if not thousands, of employees, there are steps that can be taken to move the enterprise further along the road to being a truly accountable entity.

First, the appealing mission statement hanging in the lobby is not enough. The organization must have working standards for accountability that are known to all who work there, and that are *enforced*. The woods are full of healthcare organizations that talk a great game and then end up under indictment; theories and principles and standards that are not employed in day-to-day work might as well not exist.

Furthermore, in accordance with the emerging principles of quality improvement, standards should serve as a *floor*, not a ceiling. At no time can an organization and its leaders say, "Well, we've reached this level; that's enough." We know, again, from quality improvement studies, that standing still leads almost immediately to backsliding. The bar needs to be set ever higher, and constant monitoring of how well the organization is doing in meeting its professed standards is essential.

Second, as has been widely discussed in the literature of many fields, a culture of accountability abjures finger-pointing and blame-fixing, and rather develops *positive responses* to reports of errors and problems. Going back to the children playing baseball and the broken window, we need to understand that the psychology of a punitive culture encourages covering up of mistakes and denial of responsibility. There is an enormous difference between a *blame* culture ("you blew it – you're fired!") and an *improvement* culture ("let's see what went wrong here, and how we can prevent it from happening again"). Not only will an improvement culture make things better; it will make the organization a much more attractive place to work.

Third, a culture of accountability encourages reporting of problems, because people are not in fear of punishment. Two forms of punishment are rife in a punitive culture: punishment of the person who commits the misdeed, and, even more sad, punishment of the person who reports it. Shooting the messenger of bad tidings is an old human habit, but it is utterly inappropriate in a healthcare setting, where lives are on the line. In a culture of accountability, those who identify problems and (preferably) their systemic sources should be celebrated for seeking to improve the quality of performance.

Fourth, no one should be immune from consequences. Providing indemnification against litigation for trustees or executives is commonplace and probably appropriate; providing indemnification for self-dealing, conflicts of interest, malfeasance, and harm to patients is not. At the very least, standards for membership on the board or in executive positions should include immediate removal for misbehavior, without concomitant lavish financial compensation. Any board that seeks to hire an executive who demands absolute financial and professional indemnification should think twice.

Furthermore, the "buddy system" through which healthcare executives have traditionally protected their own, no matter what they have done, should end. If someone has made an error in judgment, it should not ruin her career; however, if there has been gross misbehavior, the time is past when that executive should be protected by her peers with the gift of another lucrative leadership position. Financial irresponsibility, personal profiteering, accounting fraud, and personal misbehavior do hurt patients; equally important, they hurt the organization and all of healthcare. The public and the press do not discern technical details among hospitals, clinics, or health plans; what one does tars all with the same brush.

Fifth, public accountability is essential. Healthcare providers and plans have long argued that they are honest and above board and that their current standards are acceptable because otherwise they would be sued by the ever-hungry plaintiffs' bar. At the same time, they argue that they cannot reveal details of management or clinical mistakes because they will be sued by the ever-hungry plaintiffs' bar. Whatever one does in healthcare, one can always cite the lawyers as the reason for secrecy or laissez-faire management.

It would seem that one appealing way to prevent frivolous lawsuits and aggravation from attorneys is to be *transparent* in all of the organization's doings. Go beyond the current, largely indecipherable annual report to a broader reporting of ethics and accountability processes, problems encountered, and responses undertaken. Admit mistakes early and openly. Admit wrongdoing and what has been done to address its consequences and repeat its recurrence. Pull back the black curtain from what we do within the secret executive chamber and tell the community what is going on. The odds are that the number of lawsuits will diminish while community support grows.

Sixth, the accountable organization knows that there is no greater protection than being trusted and being worthy of it. Wall Street will have its say; the lawyers will have their say; the payers will have their say; the public will have its say. But in the end, nothing can replace being seen as honest. In the film "A Man for All Seasons," which tells the story of Sir Thomas More, who was executed by Henry VIII for refusing to accede to the king's first divorce, a conversation takes place between the king and Sir Thomas. More, desperate not to displease his king, but steadfast in his religious beliefs, asks why his opinion is so important, when all the nobles of England have already agreed to the dissolution of the marriage. The king replies: "Because you are honest; and not only that, you are *known* to be honest." Sir Thomas More was beheaded, and went willingly to the executioner's block, secure in his faith; King Henry VIII died of syphilis, having never produced a surviving male heir for his throne, which soon enough was occupied by the daughter of one of the wives he had ordered killed. History has made it clear who was saint and who was sinner.

We live in a society where accountability has been made elusive by those who do not think it is important – or, rather, who do not think it is important for *them*. But accountability is the heart and soul of healthcare. With it, leaders and their organizations can weather any storm; without it, the consequences will be far worse than what any leader can envision. Broken windows can be replaced; broken promises cannot.

REFERENCES

Ackman, D., 2003. "Feds charge Scrushy with life of crime," *Forbes*, November 5, Internet edn.

Appleby, J., 2003. "Tenet to pay $54M to settle disputed surgery case." *USA Today* August 7, Internet edn. 1B

Associated Press, 2003. "Ex-Enron employees target execs' bonuses." *Detroit Free Press* July 24, Internet edn.

Barret, D., 2002. "WorldCom settlement includes fine, ethics training for executives." *International Herald Tribune* November 27, Internet edn.

Burns, G., 2002. "Scandals shake faith in big business." *Chicago Tribune* July 28, section 1:1.

Canfield, D., 2003. "The real bottom line." *Modern Healthcare*, June 23: 50

Downey, M., 2003. "Hey, Sammy, don't take it so personally." *Chicago Tribune* June 19 section 4:1

Farrell, G., 2003. "Hunt is on for notebook that Scrushy denies exists." *USA Today* June 12

Friedman, E., 2001. "The butler did it." *Health Forum Journal* **44(4)**: 5–7

Galloro, V., 2003. "HealthSouth vs. everybody." *Modern Healthcare* August 4: 8

Hays, C., 2004. "Stewart sentenced to 5 months in prison for lying to investigators" *The New York Times*, July 16, Internet edn.

Hill, P., 2004. "WorldCom founder indicated in fraud," *Washington Times*, March 3, Internet edn.

Kaiser Daily Health Policy Report, 2003. "Individual Tenet hospitals, not parent company, should be sued for allegedly upcoding, Tenet attorneys say" June 11, Internet edn.

Lee, D., and R. White, 2002. "Tenet's stock hammered on news of probe." *Los Angeles Times* November 1, Internet edn.

Mollenkamp, C., 2003. "Accountant tried in vain to expose HealthSouth fraud." *The Wall Street Journal* May 20: A1

Parker, K., 2003. "Eat, drink, smoke, and then sue." *Chicago Tribune* July 23

Reuters News Service, 2002. "Judge OKs bonus for 1,700 at Enron." *Chicago Tribune*, April 17 section: 1: 19.

　　2003. "HealthSouth paid auditors for janitorial work-report." Private Internet communication June 11

Salant, J., 2002. "After Enron scandal, ethics is in again." *Duluth News Tribune*, October 31 Internet edn.

Stafford, M., 2002. "Druggist gets 30 years for diluting." *Chicago Sun-Times*, December 6: 34

Vrana, D., and R. D.White, 2003. "Tenet to pay $54 million in surgery scandal." *Los Angeles Times* August 6 Internet edn.

Part II

Case studies of mistakes in healthcare management

Chapters 7–14 include case studies with commentaries that reflect the complexities and implications of management mistakes. The cases, written by Frankie Perry, reveal the diversity of special interests, the competing values, and the moral conflicts that challenge healthcare managers. Perhaps most importantly these management errors provide evidence of the need for an *organizational culture* that acknowledges, examines, and learn from mistakes, so that fewer are made.

7

Medical errors: Paradise Hills Medical Center

Paradise Hills Medical Center is a 500-bed teaching hospital in a major metropolitan area of the South. It is known throughout a tri-state area for its comprehensive Oncology program and serves as a regional referral center for thousands of patients suffering from various forms of malignant disease.

Paradise Hills is affiliated with a major university and has residency programs in Internal Medicine, Surgery, Pediatrics, Obstetrics/Gynecology, Psychiatry, Radiology, and Pathology, all fully accredited by the Accrediting Commission for Graduate Medical Education. In addition, Paradise Hills also has an Oncology fellowship program, a university-affiliated nursing program, as well as training programs for radiology technicians and medical technologists. All of these teaching programs are highly regarded and attract students from across the nation.

Paradise Hills enjoys an enviable reputation throughout the area. It is known for its high-quality care, its state-of-the-art technology and its competent, caring staff. While Paradise Hills is located within a highly competitive healthcare community, it boasts a strong market share for its service area. Indeed, its oncology program enjoys a 75% market share and its patients provide significant referrals to the Surgery, Pediatrics, and Radiology programs as well.

Paradise Hills is a financially strong institution with equally strong leadership. Its past successes can, in large part, be attributed to its aggressive, visionary CEO and his exceptionally competent management staff.

But all is not as well as it seems to be at Paradise Hills. While the Oncology program still enjoys a healthy market share, it has been slowly but steadily declining from its peak of 82% two years ago. In addition, the program's medical staff are aging and some of its highest admitting physicians are contemplating retirement. The Oncology fellowship program was established a few years ago in anticipation of this, but unfortunately, thus far the graduates of this program have not elected to stay in the community. Of most concern to the CEO and his staff is the fact that the hospital's major competitor has recently recruited a highly credentialed Oncology medical group practice from the

Management Mistakes in Healthcare, ed. Paul Hofmann and Frankie Perry. Published by Cambridge University Press. © Cambridge University Press 2005.

Northeast and has committed enormous resources to strengthening its own struggling Oncology program.

Last week the Board of Trustees for Paradise Hills had its monthly meeting with a fairly routine agenda. However, during review of a standard quality assurance report, one of the trustees asked for clarification of a portion of the report indicating that twenty-two oncology patients had received radiation therapy dosages in excess of what had been prescribed for them. The board was informed that the errors had occurred due to a flaw in the calibration of the equipment. The board was also informed that the medical physicist responsible for the errors had been asked to resign his position. The question was then asked if the patients who were recipients of the excessive radiation had been told of the error. The CEO responded that it was the responsibility of the medical staff to address this issue and it was their decision that the patients not be informed of the errors. The board did not concur that the responsibility for informing the patients of the errors rested solely with the medical staff and requested that the administrative staff review the hospital's ethical responsibility to these patients, as well as its liability related to this incident, and report back to the board within two weeks.

The CEO and his management staff responsible for the Radiology Department and the Oncology program promptly met with the medical staff department chairmen for Internal Medicine and Radiology, the program medical directors for Oncology and Radiation Therapy and the attending oncologists. The CEO reported on the board discussion related to the incident and the board's request for a review of the actions taken, specifically the decision to not inform the patients affected.

The physicians as a whole agreed that the adverse effects of the accidental radiation overdose on the patients were unknown. Therefore, they argued the patients should not be told of the incident. These are cancer patients and they don't want or need anymore bad news, the oncologists argued. "Let's face it, these patients are terminal." "Informing the patients of this error will only confuse them and destroy their faith and trust in their physicians and in the hospital," they added. Furthermore, they claimed, informing the patients of the errors might unnecessarily frighten them to the extent that they might refuse further treatment and that would be even more detrimental to them. Besides, argued the physicians, advising the patients of potential ill effects just might induce these symptoms through suggestion or excessive worry. Every procedure has its risks, insisted the chairman for Radiology, and these patients had signed an informed consent.

Physicians know what is best for their patients, the attending oncologists maintained, and they will monitor these patients for any ill effects. The department chairman for Internal Medicine volunteered that, in his opinion, this incident is clearly a patient – physician relationship responsibility and not the business of the hospital. Besides, added the chairman of Radiology, informing the patients would "just be asking for malpractice litigation."

The medical director for the Oncology program then suggested that the Board of Trustees and the management staff "think long and hard" about the public relations impact of this incident on the Oncology program. "Do you really think patients will want to come to Paradise Hills if they think we're incompetent?" he asked. The CEO conceded that he supported the position of the medical staff in this matter and he, too, was especially concerned about preserving the image of the Oncology program, but "his hands were tied" since the board clearly considered this an ethical issue and one that would have to be referred to the hospital's Ethics Committee for its opinion.

The physicians noted that if indeed it was the subsequent recommendation of the Ethics Committee that these patients be informed, then realistically, that responsibility would rest with the patient's primary care physician and not with any of them.

The matter of the radiation overdosage to twenty-two oncology patients was referred to the medical center's Ethics Committee. Following deliberations, it was the committee's recommendation that the patients affected be informed of the errors and monitored closely for adverse effects. The medical staff and administration reviewed the committee's recommendations but the administration decided not to follow them and since the Ethics Committee is advisory in nature, it held that it was under no obligation to do so. After review, the Governing Board concurred. Its decision was based upon the fear of litigation and subsequent "bad" publicity that was certain to follow. Consequently, the patients involved were not informed of the errors. Four of the patients suffered adverse effects, the most serious being radiation burns.

Some three months later, one of the patients learned of the errors and filed a lawsuit against the hospital for fraud for withholding the medical error from her. Since the lawsuit was for fraud and not malpractice, the hospital's malpractice insurance did not provide coverage. The case was settled out of court for $300,000. The lawsuit and settlement received broad news coverage in both television and the local newspapers. As the remaining patients involved became aware of the incident, only a few chose to file lawsuits and these settled out of court for like amounts. The hospital considered itself "lucky."

The aftermath of this experience was characterized by tension among the staff who disagreed among themselves over what should have been done in this case. The nurses in the Oncology program were especially adamant in their belief that the patients should have been told immediately following the incident. In fact, there was some speculation that it might have been one of the nurses who informed the first patient of the errors. A prestigious oncology medical group practice, uncomfortable with all of the publicity and the inquiries from patients about the medical center's capabilities, began disassociating itself with Paradise Hills Medical Center and treating patients at a competing facility. Relationships between some primary care physicians and oncologists remained strained. The Oncology program suffered a moderate decline in census. Some members of the Governing Board felt they had been misdirected by administration. A general sense of mistrust was palpable throughout the Medical Center and employees and hospital staff were chagrined that they had to defend the Center to friends and family who were "shocked" at the disclosure.

Commentary

Frankie Perry

Truth telling/justice and fairness

The fundamental issue in this case seems to be one of *truth telling*. Is it not a basic tenet of all ethical relationships that individuals and organizations tell the truth? Is not this the "right" thing to do?

The physicians in this case have argued that telling the truth would cause more harm than good, that not sharing this incident with their patients is, in fact, in their patients' best interest. This, of course, assumes that the patients will never find out about the incident or that the patients will die without the incident ever coming to light. From a practical standpoint, this may indeed be the case. But upon closer examination, is this scenario likely or even probable? Sociologist John Denton reminds us that some twenty-one different hospital staff may interact with the patient in a single day (Denton 1978: 132). In a teaching hospital, that number is likely to be compounded. The prescribed and administered radiation therapy are a matter of medical record. Incident reports and quality assurance reports are also a matter of record. Is it realistic to believe that staff will not have questions about the incident and, worst-case scenario, inadvertently discuss it with an affected patient? Is it even possible with the great number of staff, physicians, and trustees who are privy to this information to maintain a "conspiracy of silence"? Is it right for the hospital to attempt to do this?

In the event that the patients or their families find out about the incident, after the fact, what then? What impact will this knowledge have on their opinions of the physicians and the hospital?

Clearly, human relationships depend on the communication of information. Without an honest sharing of information, there can be no trust. Unfortunately, not telling the entire truth in a situation usually means additional shading of the truth or outright lying when questions arise. Typically, one lie begets another and yet another. Lying is, quite simply, self-destructive behavior, for once found out, liars are no longer trusted (Thiroux 1986: 165).

In this case, lying or a withholding of the truth has enormous potential for undermining the image of the physicians and the hospital. If the knowledge of the incident is "discovered" by the patients or their families, the physicians and the hospital could be then accused of attempting to "cover-up" the incident. This could prove disastrous in the judgment of the community and in a court of law. Recent political scandals are a tragic reminder that the public will not stand for deceitfulness.

But, it could be argued that the intent here in withholding information is to protect the patients from unnecessary stress and anxiety, not unlike the "white lies" that one may use to spare someone's feelings in everyday life. Is this a fair comparison? Using the Golden Rule as a guide, if you or a loved one were the patient, would you want to know the truth about the incident? Or would you wish to be spared the anxiety?

In the assessment of Elizabeth Kubler-Ross (1969), "the important question is not should I tell the truth, but how I should tell the truth, or how should I share information, important or not, with those who are asking me questions or who need to know what the truth is" (1969: 262). Does her assessment apply here?

The patient's right to know

So do the patients in this case have a right to know about the incident, and how it may potentially affect them? A Patient's Bill of Rights, as published by the American Hospital Association (AHA), is publicly posted in Paradise Hills Medical Center. It states:

Open and honest communication, respect for personal and professional values, and sensitivity to differences are integral to optimal patient care.

Hospitals must ensure a health care ethic that respects the role of patients in decision-making about treatment choices and other aspects of their care.

The patient has the right to and is encouraged to obtain from physicians and other direct caregivers relevant, current, and understandable information concerning diagnosis, treatment and prognosis.

Except in emergencies when the patient lacks decision-making capacity and the need for treatment is urgent, the patient is entitled to the opportunity to discuss and request information related to the specific procedures and/or treatments, the risks involved, the possible length of recuperation, and the medically reasonable alternatives and their accompanying risks and benefits. *(AHA 1992a)*

How do these standards of conduct apply to the radiation therapy incident at Paradise Hills? The management team and the physicians involved must review their applicability. In light of the fact that these standards are publicly posted, their review must take into consideration the patient's and their family members' interpretation of the standards, as well.

Do patients and their families have a right to know when a medical error has occurred during the course of their treatment? It seems that the Federal government is saying "yes."

Adherence to the hospital's mission statement, ethical standards, and values statement

In late 1999, the Institute of Medicine published a report entitled *To Err is Human: Building a Safer Health System* (Institute of Medicine 1999), which claims that medical errors occurring in the nation's hospitals, clinics and physician offices account for the deaths of nearly 100,000 Americans each year. As could be expected, this report was covered extensively by the media and this in turn prompted a rapid political response. Congressional hearings, a report from the Quality Interagency Coordination Task Force titled *Doing What Counts for Patient Safety: Federal Actions to Reduce Medical Errors and Their Impact*, and a major policy speech on reducing medical errors by the president soon followed.

In his speech, President Clinton introduced a National Action Plan to reduce preventable medical errors by 50% within five years. This action plan called for:

- $20 million for the creation of a center for Quality Improvement in Patient Safety to sponsor research and education in reducing errors
- New regulations requiring all 6,000 hospital participants in the Medicare program to implement patient safety programs to reduce medical errors
- Development of a national, state-based system for reporting medical errors that includes mandatory reporting of preventable errors causing death or serious injury and voluntary reporting of other medical errors including "near misses"
- Support of legislation that protects provider and patient confidentiality without undermining existing tort remedies
- New steps to specifically reduce medication errors (Clinton 2000).

This National Action Plan signals governmental intervention in a domain that previously has been notorious for "policing its own" and where medical errors have been held in secret for fear of malpractice litigation and where those committing medical errors were blamed and punished and the prevailing standard for prevention of medical errors was to educate those involved in the hope that such errors would not happen again.

In an attempt to change what some have called a "conspiracy of silence," the IOM and the Quality Interagency Coordinating Task Force recommended further action, including:

- Health plans involved in the Federal Employees Health Benefits Program must implement patient safety programs by 2001
- Employers should incorporate patient safety performance into their healthcare purchasing decisions
- Periodic re-licensing and re-examination of physicians and nurses by state boards should include knowledge and competence in patient safety practices
- Healthcare organizations should have a goal of continually improved patient safety
- Proven medication safety practices should be implemented by healthcare organizations

- Accrediting bodies such as Joint Commission on Accreditation of Healthcare Organizations (JCAHO) and others should review organizational efforts to minimize errors and promote patient safety
- Computerized medical records should be implemented that are integrated with drug ordering and administrative systems (Quality Interagency Coordination Task Force 2000).

For healthcare providers, perhaps the most disconcerting of these recommendations is the mandatory reporting of medical errors to patients and their families. No responsible healthcare professional will argue with the need for strategies to reduce medical errors and provide assurances for patient safety. But the notion of placing the organization and/or its staff at risk for malpractice litigation gives one pause.

Yet, in the President's policy address he stated: "People should have access to information about a preventable medical error that causes serious injury or death of a family member, and providers should have protections to encourage reporting and prevent mistakes from happening again (Clinton 2000)." Is it reasonable to believe that this is possible – and more to the point, is the fear of litigation sufficient justification for withholding the truth from those affected by medical error? (Clinton 2000).

In fact, Kraman and Hamm (1999) argue that honesty may be the best policy in risk management. In their article in the *Annals of Internal Medicine*, they cite a study that found that of 127 families who sued their healthcare providers after perinatal injuries, 42% were motivated by suspicion of a cover-up or revenge.

Kraman and Hamm (1999) reported on the experiences of one Veterans Affairs Medical Center that implemented a policy of full disclosure of medical errors to patients and families in the presence of a family attorney, if the family so desired. The Medical Center initiated this practice because staff believed it was the "right thing to do." They also found that this honest approach resulted in unanticipated financial benefits to the Medical Center when lower-cost settlements began replacing higher-cost litigation.

Professional codes of ethical conduct

Do the existing professional codes of ethical conduct promulgated by the professional organizations and associations representing physicians, healthcare executives, and hospitals require that the incident be fully disclosed to the patients?

Excerpts from the Code of Medical Ethics and Current Opinions of the Council on Ethical and Judicial Affairs published by the American Medical Association (AMA) state:

A physician shall deal honestly with patients and colleagues, and strive to expose those physicians deficient in character or competence, or who engage in fraud or deception. *(AMA 1994: Preamble, II)*

The patient has the right to receive information from physicians and to discuss the benefits, risks and costs of appropriate treatment alternatives. Patients should receive guidance from their physicians as to the optimal course of action. Patients are also entitled to obtain copies or summaries of their medical records, to have their questions answered, to be advised of potential conflicts of interests that their physicians might have, and to receive independent professional opinions. *(AMA 1993: I)*

Among the statements in the American College of Healthcare Executives' (ACHE) Code of Ethics are:

The health care executive shall conduct all personal and professional activities with honesty, integrity, respect, fairness, and good faith in a manner that will reflect well on the profession. *(ACHE 1995: Section I, B)*

The health care executive shall assure the existence of a process that will advise patients or others served of the rights, opportunities, responsibilities, and risks regarding available health care services. *(ACHE 1995: Section II, A, 4)*

The AHA's *Ethical Conduct for Health Care Institutions* states, in part:

Health care institutions by virtue of their role as health care providers, employers, and community health resources have special responsibilities for ethical conduct and ethical practices that go beyond meeting minimum legal and regulatory standards. Their broad range of patient care, education, public health, social services, and business functions is essential to the health and well-being of their communities. These roles and functions demand that health care organizations conduct themselves in an ethical manner that emphasizes a basic community service orientation and justifies the public trust. *(AHA 1990: Introduction)*

The Governing Board of the institution is responsible for establishing and periodically evaluating the ethical standards that guide institutional policies and practices. The Governing Board must also assure that its own policies, practices, and members comply with both legal and ethical standards of behavior. The CEO is responsible for assuring that hospital medical staff, employees, and volunteers understand and adhere to these standards and for promoting a hospital environment sensitive to differing values and conducive to ethical behavior (AHA 1990: Introduction).

While the language in these ethical standards is somewhat general, the standards do provide guidance for those wrestling with this ethical dilemma. As professionals, each physician and executive must determine if her actions are consistent with their respective ethical standards.

The AHA's *Ethical Conduct for Health Care Institutions* clearly delineates the ethical responsibilities of the Governing Board and the CEO, lending credence to the argument that ethical matters involving patient–physician relationships are indeed the "business of the hospital."

Understanding the medical staff perspective

It is not surprising, however, that the physicians involved in this case would feel otherwise. A basic understanding of the factors that contribute to the medical staff orientation helps to explain why physicians adamantly protect what they consider to be their professional province.

Typically, it is the physician who enjoys the supreme position in the hospital organizational hierarchy. It is the physician who generally establishes and maintains the rules that regulate most patient care in the hospital, and it is only through the physician that the patient can access the healthcare system. Herbert Blumer (1969) suggests that all organizations "represent the application of somebody's definition of what the organization should be." It is the physician who sets the standards for patient care and who defines illness (1969: 58). The physician is granted the authority to define illness because she possesses "a body of knowledge that defines and constructs the roles to be played in the context of the institution" (Berger and Luckmann 1967: 67). Roles make it possible for institutions to exist. By virtue of the role the physician plays, she is inducted into specific areas of knowledge, not only in the narrower cognitive sense but also in the sense of norms, values, and even emotions. This knowledge may become so internalized that the physician considers the role "an inevitable fate for which [he/she] may disclaim responsibility." "I have no choice in the matter, I have to act this way because of my position" (Berger and Luckmann 1967: 76).

Physicians learn their roles through a complex *socialization process* that begins when they enter medical school. The rigors and expense of medical school, the admission requirements, the protégé system, and the collegial bonds of the medical profession all reflect occupational socialization. Upon completion of medical school, the symbolic universe of the physician includes elaborate rights, obligations, standard practices, and a role-specific vocabulary. The physician is now socialized to play her role as definer of reality for the patient (Berger and Luckmann 1967: 91).

The effects of this socialization on the moral reasoning of medical students is reflected in a study conducted by Herbert, Meslin, and Dunn at the University of Toronto and published in the *Journal of Medical Ethics* in 1992. Their research instrument presented four clinical vignettes, and respondents were asked to list the ethical issues in each: the study assumes that physicians must *recognize issues* before they can *behave appropriately*. Students in all four medical school years participated in the research project. The first-year students completed the survey during their medical school orientation. The fourth-year students identified far fewer ethical issues than the first-year students. The researchers concluded that "these studies show[ed] a disturbing pattern; the ethical sensitivity of medical students seems to decrease with more time in medical school. Is this the consequences of medical socialization and is it harmful?" they asked (Herbert, Meslin, and Dunn 1992: 142–147).

In any discussion of the role of the physician, some attention must be given to professionalism. Critical components of professionalism include *autonomy* and *self-regulation*, and the source, structure, and characteristics of professionalism place professionals in a position of dominance. Professionalism is considered by many as the ultimate in occupational status and the physician is the prototype of professionalism (Friedson 1970: 185). There are some who will argue that the physician's position of dominance is justified. After all, they say, physicians must make life and death decisions. Advocates of patient self-determination claim that physician dominance is detrimental. But the greatest challenge to the physician's dominant role in healthcare has been *managed care*. At Paradise Hills, the physicians have not yet experienced the prevalence of managed care that exists in other parts of the country.

Given the occupational socialization and the professional dominance that the Paradise Hills' physicians enjoy, it is not surprising that they tend to *believe* that matters of patient care fall strictly within their domain.

The hospital management's role and responsibility

What is the hospital management's role and responsibility in this case? What is the role and responsibility specifically of the hospital CEO? Strict adherence to a literal interpretation of the standards of ethical conduct promulgated by the ACHE and the AHA as discussed earlier, would indicate that the role of the CEO in this case is indeed a burdensome one, one in which he must balance complex needs and conflicting interests. In this case, as in the fulfillment of his other duties as CEO, he has responsibilities to the Governing Board, to the institution, to the medical staff, to the employees, to the community, to the patients, to his profession and to himself.

The CEO is mandated to carry out the policies of the Governing Board, which includes assuring compliance with the ethical standards approved by the board for the practices of the institution. The CEO, likewise, is charged with the responsibility for assuring that the institution operates in ways that are consistent with its Mission Statement and its Statement of Values, assuming one exists. Indeed, Austin Ross in his book, *Cornerstones of Leadership for Health Services Executives* (1992) says: "The CEO's greatest source of support in preserving ethical conduct within the organization is the organizational mission (Ross 1992: 28)."

Partnering with the medical staff

Paradise Hills and its management staff have a strong working relationship with its medical staff. Its Oncology physicians have been especially loyal and committed to

Paradise Hills – and, in return, hospital management has provided the resources and technology needed for the physicians to practice state-of-the-art medicine. It has been a "win–win" situation for Paradise Hills. The CEO is now determined to arrive at a solution to this problem that will preserve the existing medical staff – management relationship. Not incidentally, he knows he must avoid alienating these community-based physicians whose patients are vital to the financial viability of the hospital.

It is generally accepted that leadership hospitals embrace the core belief that medical staff participation is essential to the successful operations and strategic planning of the institution. Management in such an institution enthusiastically integrates medical staff participation into its way of doing business, fosters on-going dialogue with physicians, and recognizes the medical staff as a needed resource. The CEO at Paradise Hills has worked to develop such an environment and is staunch in his resolve that the medical staff must be full and active participants in this ethical decision-making. The CEO believes that a satisfactory solution to this incident must not violate confidentiality of patient information, must not infringe upon or threaten the patient–physician relationships, and must not precipitate a lawsuit. He knows that to secure these objectives, he must work closely with the medical staff on this issue and avoid an adversarial confrontation. The physicians must be full partners in the analysis and resolution of the problem. Their voice in the proceedings must be heard and attended to. The outcome must be one in which they have been allowed to exercise some element of control.

Fortunately, the CEO at Paradise Hills is armed with the primary prerequisite to successful partnering with the medical staff: they trust him. Now, he knows that to successfully solve this ethical problem, he must be well prepared with solid facts, a well-thought-out rationale for action and a commitment and a plan to deal with all consequences of the actions taken. The CEO and the management staff must also recognize that medical errors take their toll on the physicians and other staff that may be involved. In an organizational culture that emphasizes perfection, self-reproach, and accountability, guilt can impact upon a clinician's effectiveness in future patient care. Management must, therefore, take measures to assist staff in appropriately coping with medical errors (Morreim 2000: 56).

Leadership

In this case, as in all ethical matters, the CEO has enormous leadership responsibility. It is she who is responsible for the ethical culture within the organization, implementing the standards of ethical conduct and serving as an ethical role model for staff. While clinical professionals may bring their own codes of conduct to the workplace, it is management that must set the tone for how business is conducted, how professionals interact, and how patients are served.

Bennis and Namus (1985) are clear on this point: "The leader is responsible for the set of ethics or norms that govern the behavior of people in the organization. Leaders set the moral tone" (1985: 186).

William D. Hitt in his book, *Ethics and Leadership: Putting Theory Into Practice* (1990) cites results of research studies that demonstrate that the ethical conduct of individuals in organization is influenced greatly by their leaders. Hitt says that leaders have three basic obligations:

(1) Achieve an understanding of ethics
(2) Serve as a role model in making ethical decisions
(3) Develop and implement a plan of action for promoting ethical conduct on the part of his or her staff (1990: 4).

The significance of the leader as role model should not be underestimated. Schmidt and Posner (1983) conducted studies to identify the five primary factors by rank that influence ethical conduct in organizations:

(1) Behavior of superiors
(2) Behavior of one's peers in the organization
(3) Ethical practices of one's industry or profession
(4) Society's moral climate
(5) Existence of organizational policy (1983: 35).

Ross (1992) states that: "effective leadership is still the healthcare system's best hope for anchoring ethics, values and social responsibility within organizations." He continues: "The CEO nurtures the organizational social conscience by being personally dedicated and committed to accomplishing an organizational mission based on good ethical conduct" (1992: 30).

Ethical problems are true managerial dilemma because they represent conflict between an organization's *economic performance* and its *social obligations* to parties both within and outside the organization (Hosmer 1987). This case, like all ethical problems, requires that the CEO, his management team, and the medical staff think through the consequences of their actions on multiple dimensions, using ethical analysis as well as economic and legal analysis (Hosmer 1987: 108). While the task is complex and the conflicts may appear insurmountable, Bennis and Namus (1985) remind us that: "Leaders are persons who are able to influence others; this influence helps to establish the organizational climate for ethical conduct; ethical conduct generates trust; and trust contributes substantially to the long-term success of the organization"(1985: 186).

Conclusion

The issue analysis reveals that the situation at Paradise Hills is more complicated than might at first appear. Management has the difficult task of balancing complex needs and conflicting interests. The CEO has an especially burdensome role with responsibilities to the Governing Board, to the medical staff, to the employees, to the community, and most certainly to the patients coming to this institution for care. He is charged with the responsibility for ensuring that the organization operates in ways consistent with its mission of high-quality patient care and service to the community.

In view of this mission, it can be argued that the patient's right to know and the ethical responsibility for truth telling should be paramount considerations here. But if it follows that the patients need to be told of these medical errors, the ramifications of such disclosures need to be thoroughly examined and mitigating actions planned or implemented. What are the subtle and not so subtle ramifications of disclosure of these errors to the patients involved?

Initially, it is advantageous to investigate adverse incidents quickly and thoroughly to avoid any appearance of indifference or conspiracy. Since the Paradise Hills Board signaled the need for investigation and questioned the advisability of disclosure in this case, it does not appear that timely action occurred.

Disclosure of the errors should be preceded with a well-thought-out plan of *what information* needs to be disclosed. Candid and open dialogue that invites questions and provides honest answers will promote an atmosphere of trust that will diminish the possibility of litigation. Disclosure should be made by the attending physician with nursing staff in attendance to hear the information given to the patient and to be available for the patient to ask the inevitable questions that will arise once the physician has left the room. The substance of the disclosure should then be documented in the patient's medical record.

A proactive *public relations strategy* needs to be in place to respond to inquiries from the community or from the media, should they occur. Protecting the privacy of the patients involved is an obvious priority in such communications. A brief, but honest account of the incident, the harm done, and what has been implemented to prevent reoccurrence should suffice. Any delay in responding to inquiries should be avoided so as not to create an impression of "cover-up." Without "spinning" the information, the opportunity may present itself to make known the positive quality indicators of past performance of the Oncology program. The spokesperson for the organization should be forthright, believable, and concerned.

The impact on *clinicians* of "human error" in the delivery of patient care should not be underestimated. The principle of non-maleficence is embedded in the psyche of clinicians. Within the healthcare environment, the somewhat common practice of placing blame and exacting punishment has generated additional anxiety among care-givers. Without a doubt, the firing of the physicist at Paradise Hills will have sent a strong message to the staff. Further compounding staff anxiety in this case is the fact that the patients involved are oncology patients with whom the staff have bonded over the course of their treatment time. Candid, confidential discussions with the care-givers with staff counseling as indicated should help to manage staff anxiety and assist them in coping with the situation.

There is no information in this case that indicates the competency or the past performance evaluations of the physicist. If her past performance has been without fault, then one must question the "firing" based on this one incident and the organizational culture in which it would take place. Firing practices say much about the *organizational culture* and can send a message of zero tolerance for mistakes that only generates fear and a reluctance to admit any wrongdoing. Honesty, fairness, and respect must be characteristic of the process.

Preserving management's *positive relationship with the medical staff* needs to be a high priority in this case. Keeping the medical staff informed and involved at each decision-making point, providing legal advice, making patient counseling available to those affected, committing resources to recruit a highly qualified physicist and involving the medical staff in the process will help to demonstrate management's support of the medical staff during this crisis.

Clearly, a *preventive maintenance program* needs to be in place and regularly practiced to ensure safe and proper functioning of all medical equipment at Paradise Hills. In addition, a system of checks and balances needs to be implemented that prevents reoccurrences of errors in the future.

The CEO in this case assembled the key constituents involved in this situation, with the significant exception of nursing staff. The nursing staff in this case were emotionally bonded with the patients and had the strongest opinions in support of disclosure of the errors. The head nurse of the Oncology program could have been a valuable participant in the decision-making process and could have played a significant role in the management of nursing staff conflicts regarding this issue.

The role and the effectiveness of the hospital's *Ethics Committee* should be reviewed and evaluated on a regular basis to determine if it is meeting the needs of the organization. The Ethics Committee at Paradise Hills, consistent with common practice, serves in an advisory capacity. If, however, the committee's recommendations are frequently ignored, the effectiveness of the committee is in question. The hospital Ethics Committee should be a valuable resource for management and the medical staff and it should have a powerful influence on healthcare decisions.

It is apparent that management, the medical staff, and the board at Paradise Hills all wanted to do the "right thing" and struggled with the issues surrounding the medical errors. In all probability, the board deferred to the medical staff in this case, out of fear that these highly regarded physicians would move their desirable practices to the competition. In fact, this did happen in spite of the board's deference to the medical staff.

The struggles at Paradise Hills were difficult but they can serve as a reminder to us of Martin Luther King, Jr.'s admonition: "Cowardice asks the question, 'Is it safe?' Expediency asks the question, 'is it politic?' Vanity asks the question, 'is it popular?' but, conscience asks the question, 'is it right?' And there comes a time when one must take a position that is neither safe, nor politic, nor popular, but one must take it because one's conscience tells one that it is right."

REFERENCES

American College of Healthcare Executives, 1995. (ACHE) *Code of Ethics*: Chicago: American College of Healthcare Executives

American Hospital Association, 1990. *Ethical Conduct for Health Care Institutions*: Chicago: American Hospital Association

1992. *A Patients Bill of Rights*: Chicago: American Hospital Association

American Medical Association, 1993. *Fundamental Elements of the Patient/Physician Relationship*. Chicago: American Medical Association

1994. *Principles of Medical Ethics*. Chicago: American Medical Association

Bennis, W. and B. Namus, 1985. *Leaders: The Strategies for Taking Charge*. New York: Harper Row

Berger P. L. and T. Luckmann, 1967. *The Social Construction of Reality*. Garden City, NY: Anchor Books

Blumer H., 1969. *Symbolic Interactionism, Perspective and Method*. Englewood Cliffs, NJ: Prentice-Hall

Clinton W., 2000. "Remarks by the President on medical errors." http://www.ahrq.gov/wh22200rem.htm February 2, 2000

Denton, J. A., 1978. *Medical Sociology*. Boston: Little, Brown

Friedson, E., 1970. *Professional Dominance*. New York: Atherton Press

Herbert, P. C., EM. Meslin, and EV. Dunn, 1992. "Measuring the ethical sensitivity of medical students: a study at the University of Toronto." *Journal of Medical Ethics* **18**: 142–147

Hitt, W. D., 1990. *Ethics and Leadership: Putting Theory Into Practice*. Columbus, OH: Battalle Press

Hosmer, L. T., 1987. *The Ethics of Management*. Homewood, K: Irwin

Institute of Medicine, 1999. *To Err is Human: Building a Safer Health System*. Washington, DC: Institute of Medicine and National Academy Press

Kraman, S. S. and G. Hamm, 1999. "Risk management: extreme honesty may be the best policy." *Annals of Internal Medicine* **131**(**12**): 913–967

Kubler-Ross, E., 1969. On *Death and Dying*. New York: Macmillan

Morreim, E., 2000. "Ethical imperatives of medical errors". *Healthcare Executive*, July–August: 56

Quality Interagency Coordination Task Force, 2000. "Doing what counts for patient safety: federal actions to reduce medical errors and their impact." Report of the Quality Interagency Coordination Task Force February

Ross, A., 1992. *Cornerstones of Leadership for Health Services Executives.* Ann Arbor, MI: Health Administration Press

Schmidt, W. H. and B. Z. Posner, 1983 *Managerial Values in Perspective.* New York: American Management Association

Thiroux, J. P., 1986. *Ethics Theory and Practice.* New York: Macmillan

8

Nursing shortage: Metropolitan Community Hospital

Metropolitan Community Hospital (MCH) was in trouble. The nurse shortage, a problem throughout the country, had reached epidemic proportions at MCH. While all four of the other hospitals in town were experiencing nurse shortages, as well, none of these competing hospitals were facing the crisis that MCH now confronted. For the first time in her twelve-year tenure at MCH, Jane MacArthur, MCH's Chief Nurse Officer (CNO), was beginning to feel a little insecure about her position. In fact, she was updating her résumé and had begun to consider new opportunities.

MCH is a 250-bed privately owned, not-for-profit hospital located in the heart of a mid-size city on the East Coast. The four other hospitals in town range from 200–400 beds and include an investor-owned hospital (part of a national chain), a county hospital, a Catholic hospital (part of a regional network), and an additional privately owned community hospital. All of these facilities had been waging serious competition for the limited number of nurses within the geographic area and it seemed as if no matter what strategies MCH employed, or how many resources it committed to the task, it was clearly losing to the competition. In the past two years, the five area hospitals had engaged in a bidding war in terms of salaries, sign-on bonuses, and benefits such as relocation expenses, tuition reimbursement, domestic partner healthcare coverage, and the like. MCH simply could not match the apparent deep pockets of some of its competitors. The nurse turnover rate at MCH had reached 25% as nurses left MCH to take more lucrative positions at competing hospitals.

MCH's geographic location was an additional recruiting obstacle. Its urban neighbor-hood was believed to be a high-crime area and although statistics disproved this, the perception remained among the predominantly young female nurse population. Jane was aware of this perception, but because it was not supported in fact, she dismissed it as not needing her attention.

As more and more foreign nurses were recruited to MCH and as an increasingly higher percentage of agency staff were being used, the budget overrun for nurse staffing reached

Management Mistakes in Healthcare, ed. Paul Hofmann and Frankie Perry. Published by Cambridge University Press. © Cambridge University Press 2005.

record proportions. The board had become impatient with Jane's attempts at justifying this cost overrun. In the words of the board chairman: "We can no longer tolerate explanations for the problem. We need solutions for the problem."

And the problem had become more significant than just cost overruns. The nurse–patient ratio on the medical–surgical units at MCH was 1:12 and by any standard, this was considered an unacceptable level for both patient safety and quality of care. Patient and family complaints had increased dramatically over the past year. Adverse events had also increased and John Fairfield, the hospital's legal counsel who had never been one of Jane's supporters, was quick to remind the CEO and the MCH board that the source of these potential litigations was failure to remedy the nurse shortage.

Two years earlier, when Eugene Wellborn had been hired as CEO at MCH, the nurse shortage was identified as a problem but was not one high on the board's list of priorities for Eugene to tackle. In fact, the board chairman had assured Eugene that Jane MacArthur was unquestionably competent and could be relied upon to resolve the issue satisfactorily. The message was clear that Nursing took care of itself and that Jane had the full confidence of the board. In retrospect, Eugene wished he had not been so hesitant in dealing with this issue. The nurse shortage occupied a huge proportion of his daily schedule and usurped time and energy needed to spend on the hospital's other pressing agenda items. Hardly a day passed that Eugene did not have to deal with an irate patient, family member, or physician.

The nurse shortage at MCH had been the major topic of discussion at last month's general Medical Staff meeting and had been accompanied by threats of diverting patient admissions to competing hospitals if the situation did not improve immediately. Jane was quick to point out that physicians were a major part of the problem and one of the reasons she was having difficulty recruiting and retaining nurses.

The strong political clout of the medical staff had positioned it as a body to which deference was paid on questions of authority, facility planning, and patient care. Past administrations had abdicated much of their responsibilities related to patient care and seemed indifferent to issues other than the financial viability of the institution and its public image throughout the community. Attracting physicians had been a major priority in the recent past and Eugene's predecessor had spent every Wednesday afternoon on the golf course with prominent members of the Medical Executive Staff Committee.

Eugene left this kind of relationship building to Carter Sims, MCH's young, ambitious Chief Operating Officer (COO). For his part, Eugene saw his role and responsibility as CEO to focus on the external environment. He needed to develop collaborative relationships and coalitions throughout the community if MCH were to survive into the future. This was his strong belief and the mandate he had received from the board.

Nevertheless, Eugene was troubled by the powerful position of the medical staff and he agreed with Jane that the behavior of some of the physicians contributed to the exodus of nurses. He had been reluctant to confront the medical staff leadership on this issue, believing that he needed to develop a stronger relationship with the physicians before taking on such an adversarial role.

To the nursing staff at MCH, this administrative posture clearly reflected that nurses were the "hired help" and should do no more than "follow the orders of the physicians." In this environment, the physicians in large part had become accustomed to behaving in an autocratic – and, in some instances, a disrespectful – manner to the nurses. John Fairfield had on more than one occasion cautioned Eugene about the legal implications of acts that he believed bordered on harassment. These incidents had fueled hostile outbursts between Jane and the Chief of the Medical Staff who she believed turned a blind eye to inappropriate behavior on the part of physicians.

In some ways, Jane's management style mirrored the autocratic, disrespectful approach to the nursing staff favored by some physicians. Jane, on the other hand, saw herself as a benevolent dictator, always ready to do battle in defense of her "underlings." The nursing staff resented both of these higher authorities. Behind Jane's back, they referred to her as "the general." Some of the physicians fared less well in the name-calling. It was the nurses' opinion that "they did all of the work and received none of the rewards." They had no authority or control over their work and no participation in the decision-making surrounding patient care. They received no recognition or respect for the physically and emotionally stressful work they were expected to perform without regard to personal or professional preferences. Their work schedules were frequently modified, overtime was often required, and they were arbitrarily pulled from their work units to float to an unfamiliar, understaffed area of the hospital.

The informal leaders among the nursing staff had begun to talk about "organizing." Some of them had complained to Carter Sims, but it seemed that the administration's answer to the nurses' complaints was to "throw money at the problem." In fact, Carter Sims was overheard to say: "If we pay them enough, they'll be happy." And that did seem to be the case with the foreign nurses who MCH recruited. They seemed willing to tolerate the unpleasant working conditions if the pay was good. This difference of opinion created resentment between the foreign recruits and the American nurses who believed the foreigners were encouraging this unfair treatment by allowing themselves to be exploited. This resentment spawned a lack of cooperation and tension among the nurses that could not help but be observed by patients. Eugene knew it was just a matter of time before news of this disruptive environment at MCH reached the community, and he would hear about it at the Rotary Club.

The only patient care units in MCH that were peaceful and operated efficiently were Emergency, the Operating Room and Intensive Care. The physician–nursing coalitions on these patient care units made them "untouchables." Both Jane and the attending physicians knew better than to antagonize the skilled, experienced, and confident nurses who were considered irreplaceable by the medical directors of these units. Indeed, the nurses on these units were considered more competent and more valuable than some of the attending physicians whose patients were treated there.

As Eugene pondered the situation at MCH, he knew he must take action and he knew it was not going to be pleasant.

Commentary

Trudy Land

Healthcare is one of the most complex sectors of society, with multiple variables that present both challenges and opportunities. An issue of critical importance facing today's healthcare leaders is the work force shortage. According to Janet F. Quinn (2002), "The nurse shortage is one of the most serious threats to quality care facing the healthcare system" (2002: 3). In order to deal with this significant issue, it is imperative that an organization examine its performance, identify the root causes of problems, have the courage to make changes, determine the best procedures and processes, and develop effective strategies.

Failure Analysis

MCH is in trouble. Its nursing shortage has reached epidemic proportions. The mission of the hospital is to provide excellent patient care and to meet the healthcare needs of the community. In order to fulfill this mission, the organization must have a cohesive and collaborative team of physicians, clinical staff, and support staff. The nurse shortage and high turnover rate are major problems at MCH and if a plan is not immediately implemented to correct the situation the survival of MCH is in question. MCH is facing a crisis and is losing to the competition in its community.

There are many issues this organization is facing on both micro- and macro-levels involving employees, the board, executive leadership, the medical staff, and the community that are contributing to this crisis:

- Why is MCH so organizationally dysfunctional?
- What management mistakes have occurred?
- How could these mistakes have been avoided?
- What steps could be taken in this organization to prevent these kinds of mistakes in the future?

Mismanagement at MCH involves a number of areas and actions on the part of a number of persons. The mistakes contributing most to the current crisis at MCH include:

(1) The CEO's *passive acceptance of the board directives* without supporting evidence

(2) The CEO's failure to conduct an *internal operations assessment* at MCH

(3) The CEO's failure to *critically evaluate the performance of the existing management team* at MCH

(4) The *disregard of the hospital's mission* by the governance and the management of MCH while they pursued lesser priorities

(5) Failure of the leadership of the organization to deal with *disruptive physician behaviors*

(6) Allowing the organizational culture to *deteriorate into one of negativism.*

The foundation of an organization is its *people.* If the right people cannot be recruited and retained, the system will not be viable and will not achieve positive outcomes in terms of employee, patient, and physician satisfaction, clinical results, financial targets, and business plans. The development of an organizational culture that focuses on its employees and their participation in decision-making, strives for excellence, acknowledges mistakes and opportunities for improvement, takes risks, and continually analyzes its processes to prevent errors, will thrive in today's healthcare environment.

Almost every institution in this country is facing the dilemma of workforce shortages. There are multiple reasons and causal factors for this problem, including:

- Insufficient number of people entering or interested in nursing and other clinical healthcare professions
- Aging labor pool and teaching faculty
- Aging general population with growing medical needs
- Women who are entering more lucrative careers with less stress and less risk and liability
- Women who have left these professions and have decided to remain at home with their families
- Public image of the professions
- Supply and demand in economic terms
- Lack of competitive wages and benefits
- Non-supportive work environments that do not provide recognition, education, and advancement opportunities, and participation in decision-making
- Healthcare leadership that does not recognize the extent of the problem and does not take proactive measures and immediate action
- Poor nurse–staffing ratios
- Negative or disruptive physician behavior in relationship to other professionals.

According to Wolf (2001: 14), "The combined pressures of a shrinking work force, an aging population, changing social attitudes toward work, financial constraints, and public perception of healthcare have contributed to a growing personnel problem for healthcare organizations across the country." Wolf also states: "Though the nursing shortage has received much attention, labor shortages are not limited to any one occupation in the healthcare field. Healthcare organizations are also facing a decreasing applicant pool of caregivers in general, including pharmacists, technicians, technologists, and therapists"(2001: 15).

In this case, the critical operational situation at MCH involves many constituencies and a system that is deteriorating on both macro- and micro-levels. What has contributed to this situation at MCH, and what can be done to resolve problems of this magnitude?

Failure to validate the board's analysis of priorities

When Eugene Wellborn was hired as CEO at MCH, the nurse shortage was not on the board's list of top priorities. This information was communicated to Eugene by the board chairman who also voiced the board's complete confidence in Jane MacArthur, MCH's CNO, to deal with the nurse shortage. It was an initial management mistake for Eugene to accept this assessment without question. As the CEO, Eugene had a responsibility to gather the necessary information to adequately assess the problem, to determine the root cause or causal factors of the problem, to communicate this information to the board, and to develop with his management team strategies to resolve the problem. These are steps taken by effective leaders.

Failure to conduct assessment of internal operations

As a newly hired CEO, Eugene had the task of developing relationships of *trust and integrity with key constituencies*. But he was also responsible for assessing the organization as a *system*; obtaining sufficient, accurate, and reliable data, sharing this information with key stakeholders, and preparing the decision-makers. Eugene admits his hesitancy in dealing with the nursing shortage. He faced the political pressures of a new position, his board's approval, as well as the risk of challenging the board's priorities. Eugene also had serious problems with medical staff relationships at MCH, and with its community image. Eugene's acceptance of the board's priorities and his lack of adequate information, preparation, and thorough evaluation of the situation are primary causes of management mistakes in this case.

Clearly, the working relationship between Eugene and his board chairman does not appear to be one that supports the needs of the organization. In their book, *Practical Governance*, Tyler and Biggs (2001: 25), identified five universal truths for board chairs:

(1) Lead the board
(2) Cultivate an effective working relationship with the CEO
(3) Mentor others on the board
(4) Be decisive and move the board to action
(5) Walk the straight and narrow.

Tyler and Biggs (2001: 13) also identified five universal truths for CEOs:
(1) Communicate effectively and frequently
(2) Avoid suddenly springing information on the board
(3) Recognize that he or she serves at the pleasure of the board
(4) Be a visionary and inspire the board with that vision
(5) Take calculated risks.

Eugene believed that his primary responsibility, as mandated by the board, was to focus on the external environment and to build collaborative relationships with the community. Although these are important functions and roles for CEOs, the internal organization cannot be ignored and must remain a primary focus as well. Eugene was aware that the nurse shortage was a major problem. He knew that the nurse turnover rate, percentage of agency staff and the number of foreign nurses, and the budget variance for nurse staffing required immediate attention. He was also aware of the board's frustration with the nursing issue, the existing employee dissatisfaction, the powerful position of the medical staff, and the disruptive behavior of some physicians. Although Eugene was aware of these significant problems, he continued to believe that his role was to focus on the external environment, as mandated from the board.

As stated by Tyler and Biggs(2001: 21) regarding the CEO's role, "More than anyone else on your board or on your staff, you have, or should have, a 'big picture' understanding of your organization and its need to flourish." Eugene, in this case, ignored the "big picture" assessment of the nursing shortage and failed to present this information and the seriousness of the situation to the board. This is a fundamental responsibility of the CEO.

Eugene had not made it a personal priority to establish the positive and effective relationships with the board and medical staff that would allow him to confidently communicate challenging information, deal with difficult issues, and confront problems with the key groups. It appears that Eugene fears any risk of confrontation with these influential groups. According to Tyler and Biggs (2001: 21), "Taking risks is risky. But we believe not taking risks is even riskier."

When hiring a new CEO, it is necessary for the board to establish a trusting relationship through effective communication early on. Development of a list of priorities for the organization is the responsibility of the CEO working in partnership with the board, medical staff, and the management team. Information from a comprehensive assessment of the organization and the external environment is required to determine how priorities are established and how strategies and action plans are developed to achieve desirable goals and outcomes. This collaborative assessment did not occur at MCH. The board had established the priorities in isolation and had evaluated the senior nursing executive's ability to handle the nursing shortage without a proper assessment. The board's role is to set policy and function on the macro-level, it is the CEO's role to manage the operations of the hospital in a manner consistent with policy.

When Eugene recognized the seriousness of the situation at MCH and his own reluctance and lack of confidence in dealing with the board, the medical staff, and the nursing leadership, it might have been helpful for him to seek confidential advice from those outside the organization. This counsel and guidance, if he had established professional networks with mentors and colleagues, could have assisted Eugene in developing a plan for approaching each issue.

Failure to evaluate the performance of the management team

The next apparent management error in this case is the failure to assess and develop a *competent executive team*. A competent executive team, that can trust its members and is held accountable for responsibilities, is absolutely necessary for the effective operations of MCH. Failure to assess and provide feedback to each team member and hold each individual responsible for his or her duties is an act of omission on the part of the CEO. When Eugene arrived, it should have been one of his first priorities to assess the level of competence of Jane MacArthur and Carter Simms, among others. Eugene accepted without question the board's evaluation of Jane's competence in resolving the nursing situation and he accepted the board chairman's judgment that nursing took care of itself. These statements should have been red flags for Eugene; however, he remained focused on the mandate he received from the board, and ignored the broader organizational consequences of the nurse shortage.

As the CEO, Eugene was obligated to evaluate the team, establish expectations, clearly define roles and responsibilities, develop the individuals as a team, hold the members accountable, and take the necessary actions to resolve personnel problems. He did not fulfill this important role, which could have helped to prevent the nursing situation from becoming the current crisis.

Jane MacArthur, MCH's CNO, has been with the organization for twelve years and is aware of the nurse shortage and the behavior of the physicians. At the root cause of the nursing situation is Jane's leadership style, which she has described as "benevolent dictatorship," but which mirrors the autocratic, disrespectful approach to the nursing staff favored by some physicians. The nursing staff feel that they do all the work and receive no respect or recognition. They do not believe they have any authority or control over their work and no participation in decision-making surrounding patient care.

It was Eugene's responsibility to assess this information in terms of Jane's managerial style, perceptions of her leadership approach and the consequences, and how her style fitted within the executive team and the organization. Does Jane have the necessary knowledge and skills to perform in her position? She apparently does not have the trust and respect of the staff or the interpersonal skills to develop and maintain a team. If she received constructive feedback in an evaluation, could she change her style or would she choose to correct her style? Could she change the perceptions of the staff? Could this change occur quickly enough to recruit and retain staff? Jane is beginning to feel insecure about her position and is starting to consider new opportunities. The board is becoming impatient regarding her explanations of expense variances. Jane does not have a good relationship with the Chief of Staff. Should Jane resign or should her employment be terminated?

As stated in the Executive Summary, *Best Practices in Retention* of The Founders Council of The Advisory Board Company, (2000): "Although compensation and benefits packages are the most common strategy used to improve general employee retention, employee satisfaction is more closely linked to organizational culture, administrative communication and management practices." MCH has a *negative culture*, and this is one of the root causes of this dysfunctional system. Jane must be held accountable for her role in contributing to this culture.

Failure to respect and support MCH's mission

Perhaps the most significant and the most serious area of mismanagement in this case is the failure of both the board and the CEO to respect and to adhere to the mission of MCH – providing cost-effective patient care and meeting the healthcare needs of the community.

Eugene was aware that past administrations had abdicated much of their responsibilities related to patient care and had seemed indifferent to issues other than the financial viability of the institution and its public image throughout the community. The obvious need to restore patient care as paramount within the organization was a major omission on the part of both Eugene and the board.

Tyler and Biggs (2001: 35) enumerate five universal truths for boards, and state that boards must:
(1) demonstrate commitment to the job
(2) set policy, not oversee day-to-day operations
(3) guard against self-dealing
(4) take corrective action when necessary
(5) stay focused on community needs.
The MCH board has lost sight of its primary focus and has misdirected its new CEO. Eugene, believing he "serves at the pleasure of the board" has not challenged the board's direction and MCH is suffering as a result of this mismanagement.

While the board was aware of the operational problems at MCH, it seemed incapable of other than linear thinking in the prioritizing of the critical activities necessary for MCH's survival in its marketplace. Given the failure of the previous administration to act in concert with the mission of the hospital, it begs a number of questions of the governing board. Did the board direct the previous CEO to recruit physicians to MCH at any cost, and was the current political clout of the medical staff the result? Was the direction given to both past and present administrators the consensus of the board as a whole or the opinion and point of view of an over powering board chairman?

The board's poor performance in the governance of this organization has significantly contributed to the poor performance of the organization itself. It is apparent that the board could benefit from trustee development and education as to its role and its responsibilities to evaluate organizational performance, interpret reports and data, and assess the organization's ability to fulfill its mission.

Failure to address disruptive physician behavior

In order for the board and the CEO to effectively execute their responsibilities, there must be an exchange of complete and accurate information within an environment of trust and shared values. Failure of the senior management, the medical staff leadership, and the board to deal with the inappropriate disruptive behavior of some of the physicians has had serious consequences at MCH. It has contributed to the nurse shortage, low staff morale, and most likely to the quality of patient care.

Working with physician leaders both formal (board representatives, department chairs, etc.) and informal could have assisted in balancing the power interests of the medical staff as related to authority, planning, and patient care. These physician leaders could have assisted in the recruitment and retention of medical staff and could have held the Medical Executive Committee or other appropriate medical staff authority responsible for dealing with the negative behavior of certain physicians. They could have played an active role in facilitating and promoting positive relationships among the nursing staff and physicians.

Failure to improve organizational culture

The organizational culture at MCH has been allowed to deteriorate into one of negative and counter productive attitudes and behaviors. Cultural development with a foundation of values followed and promoted in the organization is a basic responsibility of the leaders at MCH. If change is to occur at MCH, the culture must evolve in a positive way with values of trust, respect, and integrity, and with a focus on employees, physicians, and the board as integral partners in participating in organizational development and decision-making. A positive culture includes communication at all levels of the organization and management practices that demonstrate on a daily basis the value of each employee, physician, patient, family, and member of the community.

The environment at MCH is described as disruptive with unpleasant working conditions. The informal nurse leaders are talking about "organizing." The staff do not feel respected and do not feel they have control over their work or involvement in decisions regarding patient care. They are not empowered and do not feel they receive any recognition, with the exception of the nurses in the Emergency Department, Operating Room, and the Intensive Care Unit. These areas are described as "peaceful" and "efficient" due to the physician–nurse coalitions and the competency, skill, and confidence of the nurses who have control and authority within their work environment. But this is the exception. There is also the issue of the negative relationships between and among the foreign nurses and the American nurses.

The root causes of these problems can be seen in the inadequate nursing leadership and cultural development, the lack of respect within the work environment, and ineffective communication with staff. If an enriching, diverse environment that included shared governance, control over patient care and nursing practices, and respect for each professional had been created by Jane, the significant problems at MCH could have been prevented. Jane's style of leadership has not allowed or promoted the type of environment necessary to recruit and retain staff. The executive team, board, and medical staff leaders also have not provided the support or the organizational culture required for employee and patient satisfaction.

The leaders of this organization must demonstrate their willingness to listen and communicate with staff with an openness to change that will create an environment of trust and respect. They must respond immediately to disrespectful and negative behavior between members of the organization; develop a partnership with employees; and seriously follow through on the suggestions and recommendations of the staff.

Regular management rounds by teams of senior level administrators and medical staff leaders would demonstrate a sincere interest in the veritable business of the organization and a genuine commitment to the employees who are working to fulfill the organization's mission. This kind of *visibility* fosters an environment of trust, loyalty, and a commitment to shared values.

If MCH does not cultivate a new culture sustained with effective leadership, the organization will continue to deteriorate. The turnover rate will increase and recruitment efforts will fail if nurses do not perceive their leader as a nursing advocate as well as one who is knowledgeable and competent. Jane must be replaced immediately. It is Eugene's responsibility to take this action and to recruit a new nursing leader with the participation and support of staff, physicians, and the board. The selection of a new nursing leader will begin to move the environment at MCH in a positive direction.

Strategies for change

Significant and fundamental changes are required to prevent the mistakes that have occurred at MCH from recurring in the future and to transition MCH into an effective and efficient organization. In order to turn around the organization and the perceptions of MCH by professionals and the community, Eugene and the executive team, the board, and medical staff leaders must demonstrate their commitment to change MCH, and must develop strategies and action plans to make that change happen.

Eugene must enhance his communication with the board and medical staff leaders and develop relationships with them that support the open sharing of information concerning the assessment, root causes of key issues and problems, and proposed strategies for change. Although this may be a difficult process for Eugene, his survival as a CEO is contingent upon it. If Eugene can accomplish these tasks, the organization will be positioned for a better future.

As for nursing, the American Nurses Credentialing Center utilizes the "14 forces of magnetism" with other criteria in assessing applicants for magnet hospital status. The "14 forces of magnetism" summarize clearly the critical questions to be answered by MCH and the areas of focus in the development of strategies for improvement (Romano 2002: 30):

(1) *Quality of nursing leadership*: are they strong, knowledgeable advocates for the staff?

(2) *Organizational structure*: is it decentralized, with strong representation for nurses?

(3) *Management style*: do the leaders invite participation and feedback?

(4) *Personnel policies and programs*: are salaries competitive? Are staffers offered flexible schedules?

(5) *Professional models of care*: are nurses given responsibility and authority?

(6) *Quality of care*: is it an organizational priority?

(7) *Quality improvement*: are nurses involved?

(8) *Consultation and resources*: are there adequate human resources?

(9) *Autonomy*: are nurses allowed independent judgment?

(10) *Community and the hospital*: is there a strong presence in the community?

(11) *Nurses as teachers*: are nurses permitted – and expected – to incorporate teaching in all aspects of practice?

(12) *Image of nursing*: is the work of nurses characterized as essential by other members of the healthcare team?

(13) *Interdisciplinary relationships*: is a sense of mutual respect exhibited among all disciplines?

(14) *Professional development*: is significant emphasis placed on in-service education, continuing education, and career development?

These changes will require an undetermined period of time, but a plan to move the organization in the direction of magnet status is necessary for MCH's survival. A new nursing leader must demonstrate a visible commitment to change, if this leader holds forums with nursing staff – and, at the same time, Eugene holds forums with the general staff in the organization, – an openness to change will be exhibited. Throughout these team meetings, the leaders must listen to the concerns and needs of staff. Visible follow through on suggestions and recommendations will begin the process of fostering trust and respect. Involving staff and encouraging their participation in important decisions concerning their responsibilities for patient care will be the next step in the evolution of a new culture and environment at MCH.

Based on these forums and a shared governance model within nursing, problem areas will be identified and solutions developed. The support of the board and the medical staff leadership throughout the change process, and their willingness to confront the behavioral problems of physicians, will be of the utmost importance if the organization is to thrive. All constituencies must clearly understand the issues, the root causes of mistakes that have occurred, actions to prevent future mistakes, and their participation in problem resolution.

An environment of caring and compassion must be developed. MCH has a history of conflicts and problems, and it must now prove that it is evolving internally and externally as a different organization. A simultaneous effort to effect change on all levels of the MCH system must be made. There must be a commitment by all parties to improve MCH. It is on the verge of losing more staff, having further difficulty in recruiting staff and physicians, and suffering a serious negative public image, all of this makes MCH vulnerable to closing its doors, merging with one of its competitors, or being acquired by another system. A turnaround in all areas of operations is required for survival.

With a unified effort and a focus on the "14 forces of magnetism," nurses and other staff members within the organization may be retained. The organization can then begin the process of recruitment while it is continuing its transition. Recruitment and retention will decrease agency costs and provide the necessary resources to compete with other hospitals in salaries, wages, and benefits. As the nurse–patient ratio reaches an acceptable level according to best-demonstrated practices, and is agreed upon by the shared governance group of nurses, employee and patient satisfaction will increase and quality outcomes will improve. Patient and family complaints will decrease, along with adverse outcomes and potential litigation.

If MCH is to distinguish itself in the community and with its competitors, it has to *demonstrate excellence* in its culture, in the delivery of patient care, and in comparative quality indicators. The leaders of MCH will have to constantly communicate key messages that prove that the organization is changing and is improving all operations. Building relationships, networking, and communicating with all constituencies regarding the progress of MCH will be critical to its success.

What more can be done to prevent future mistakes at MCH, and to move the organization in a positive direction? The governance of MCH needs to be in the hands of skilled and knowledgeable trustees with the necessary competencies. Based on established criteria to meet the needs of the board and hospital, diverse and representative members must be selected. The board must have an effective chairman who can lead the members and the organization according to the hospital's agreed strategic direction.

In "Putting all The Pieces Together: The Complete Board Needs the Right Mix of Competencies," Bader and O'Malley (2002) list competencies in three categories

(1) *Universal competencies*: personal characteristics that all members should possess, such as commitment to the mission, integrity, and ability to make objective decisions.

(2) *Collective competencies*: qualifications that at least some trustees should have, such as financial and business acumen and executive-level business experience.

(3) *Desirable competencies*: needs the board hopes to fill, such as greater gender and ethnic diversity, or expertise in emerging fields such as information technology (IT) consumerism(2002: 8).

If the board members are not fulfilling their responsibilities and are not providing effective leadership, they must be replaced. With board members meeting the defined competencies, a thorough and comprehensive orientation is required. This orientation includes the members' roles and responsibilities and the mission, vision, and values statements of MCH which need to be developed and clearly understood and communicated by the leaders. Other programs and information that must be understood by board members include: the compliance program, the strategic plan, quality outcomes, community needs assessments, financial reports, operational performance indicators, regulatory survey results, patient, physician, and employee satisfaction surveys, and other material appropriate to the members' roles.

After the board members and chairman have been oriented to their roles and are effectively governing the organization, continuing education is necessary through conferences and retreats. Education is determined based on the board's annual or more frequent self-assessments. These evaluations focus on crucial governance issues and allow the members to interact and communicate, forming stronger working relationships.

Getting the right people on board

Jim Collins, in his national bestseller, *Good To Great* (2001), tells us that: "executives who ignited the transformations from good to great [companies] did not first figure out where to drive the bus and then get people to take it there ... they first got the right people on the bus (and the wrong people off the bus) and then figured out where to drive it" (2000: 41).

A critical step in the process to prevent future mistakes at MCH is to hire the right executive management team with the necessary *competencies and cultural fit* to manage and grow the organization. This team needs to partner with the board and medical staff in creating a positive culture, assessing MCH, developing a strategic plan, carrying out its mission of excellent patient care, establishing relationships with the community, and monitoring MCH's operational performance. The executive team members must be skilled listeners and communicators capable of cultivating relationships with all the key constituencies. They must demonstrate this behavior on a daily basis to build trust. Unless Eugene takes a leadership role in modeling this behavior, he may need to be replaced.

If MCH is to change, a new CNO must be a dynamic force in building a positive culture; recruiting and retaining staff; and partnering with employees, physicians, the board, and the community in achieving objectives of quality patient care. A *participatory style of leadership* empowering and recognizing employees will precipitate change.

Carter Sims is the young, ambitious COO at MCH. Eugene has delegated building relationships with the medical staff leadership to Carter while he focused on the external environment. It is evident in this organization that Eugene must be responsible for these key physician relationships and must clearly communicate new expectations and responsibilities of the COO position. If it is assumed that Carter has had little management experience, then Eugene must be a mentor and a coach guiding Carter. Does Carter have executive potential? Can Eugene assist Carter in being successful in his job? If the answer is "yes," then Eugene must restructure Carter's responsibilities with clear expectations and accountabilities for internal operations and departmental medical staff relations. If Carter is not capable of performing the newly assigned tasks after he has been given the opportunity to improve his management performance, it may be necessary to terminate his employment. It appears that a management leader with more experience, knowledge, and skills in being a *change agent* would assist the organization in accelerating change and managing MCH's complexity.

With an effective board and the right executive talent, MCH is now positioned to complete a comprehensive assessment of the organization's functioning; to build key relationships within and outside the organization; to develop an organizational culture of loyalty and trust; and to determine present and future strategic initiatives. These actions must be implemented *simultaneously* in order to achieve the magnitude of change necessary for MCH.

Positioning MCH for the future

The future success of MCH requires that a partnership with the medical staff be developed and continually cultivated. The medical staff at MCH has sufficient political clout and authority to cause some physicians to believe that they can behave in an autocratic and a disrespectful manner with the nursing staff. Physician leaders, in concert with management, must demonstrate an intolerance for such disrespectful behavior. Communication, listening, and role modeling are the ingredients in building a foundation of trust, and these behaviors must be nurtured among members of management and the medical staff in order to forge an effective partnership. To collaborate successfully with the medical staff, physicians must feel understood and engaged; and they must understand their roles as well as the roles of the board and administration. Physicians need to be involved in a mutually beneficial manner in operational matters, patient care issues, capital expenditure decisions, strategic planning, and medical staff recruitment. Mechanisms need to be developed for their input and to encourage their participation.

With a successful partnership of the board, medical staff leaders, and the executive team in place, the next step involves a thorough *internal assessment* of the organization and the external environment to determine action plans and strategies to improve MCH's performance. This evaluation and review of the mission, vision, and values will guide the development of the blueprint for MCH's future. The assessment must include information related to quality outcomes; patient, employee, and physician satisfaction; financial goals and results; community image; competitor data; strengths, weaknesses, opportunities, threats (SWOT), and critical issues.

In "Stewardship of the Future," Orlikoff and Totten (2000), state: "To know where its organization is capable of going, a board must be firmly grounded in where its organization is. So, the first step that every board must take is to thoroughly and honestly assess its organization's vitality and viability." The board, senior management, and medical staff leaders are responsible for this assessment and for reaching a consensus as to the present status of MCH. Once there is agreement, the leaders can move forward to the next stage of strategy development. MCH has many significant and critical issues to confront. The survivability of the organization has been threatened by poor management performance. If MCH is to survive, the root causes of problems must be recognized, analyzed, and resolved. These root causal factors and key issues must determine the priorities and strategies for MCH.

For MCH, dramatic change is necessary to turn around its present dysfunction on both macro- and micro-levels. Clearly, the board has primary responsibility and accountability for MCH's future. As stated by Orlikoff and Totten (2000): "Health care governing boards are now doubly challenged. They must lead their organizations simultaneously toward achieving today's mission even as they set strategic direction toward a future that is likely to fundamentally change the organization they now govern. As boards increasingly embrace their role as stewards of the future, they need to shift their frame of reference, always inter-preting today's focus and performance in terms of its future implications and the strategic options those implications suggest."

MCH must have stewards who can govern the organization in an effective manner. The right people have to be in the stewardship, management, and medical staff roles. Only with the right people can MCH fulfill its mission of quality patient care and service to the community. And in order to achieve quality patient care, the nurse shortage must be a board priority. According to Linda H. Aiken (Smith 2002: 59): "In hospitals with administrative support for nurses and where staff resources were adequate, outcomes for both patients and nurses were better." The benefits to MCH will be enormous when retaining staff and providing the necessary resources is a matter of course.

The key action step within the retention and recruitment strategy is attaining "magnet status" through the American Nurses Credentialing Center. Aiken states (Smith 2002: 60): "The magnet approach remains the most proven strategy to achieve improved patient and nurse outcomes" (2002: 59–60). If MCH with its new nursing leader can meet the criteria established for this designation, MCH could exponentially change its environment and the perceptions of the nurses inside and outside the organization as well as the public's and healthcare com-munity's image of the hospital. Nurses will be retained and new nurses recruited. The new CNO must be charged with the responsibility of working toward meeting the criteria for "magnet status" at MCH. A prerequisite to this designation would be a *shared governance council for nursing*, the new Chief Nurse Officer would be well advised to seek peer nominations for such a council, recognizing that tapping into the informal leadership of the nursing staff may well guarantee the council's success.

In addition, a more advanced *quality–performance improvement system* at MCH would contribute significantly to improved operations. *Performance indicators* must be developed and utilized to monitor the performance of MCH as a system, to determine areas for improvement, and to improve operations. *Best-demonstrated processes and practices* can provide guidelines to achieve quality care and services. A significant differentiation strategy for MCH should be the demonstration of excellence in patient care in comparison to its healthcare competitors. If MCH is to gain market share and develop a strategic position, objective data clearly showing its clinical performance will be necessary. Achieving high-quality outcomes and communicating these results will provide leverage for MCH to establish its place in the healthcare community.

It is therefore critical that the board, senior management, and the medical staff leaders promote and support quality improvement efforts and devote the resources to accomplish the defined goals. The focus must be on *continuous improvement* of the organization's systems and processes.

MCH also needs to address the recruitment and retention of physicians at the hospital. As with the nursing staff, physicians will want to practice at a hospital with excellent nursing care, quality outcomes, an open and trustworthy environment, and a respected administration. If MCH successfully creates this environment, physicians will remain loyal and committed to the organization and will want their patients to utilize inpatient and outpatient services. If their level of satisfaction is high, they will assist in recruiting other physicians to the medical staff.

Working successfully with physicians requires an understanding of physician mentality. Physicians tend to be results-oriented professionals with little patience for bureaucratic red tape. Establishing clear lines of communication, both formal and informal, that foster a *collegial relationship* between management and the medical staff will help to partner with physicians to resolve behavioral issues before they become disruptive.

Management visibility in patient care areas and immersion within the physician's "world within the institution" – e.g. medical staff meetings, conferences, lounge areas, etc. – will advance the notion of a medical staff–management partnership working to further the interests of the organization.

Developing collaborative relationships and partnerships with *community groups*, as with employees and physicians, is also critical for MCH's survival. Establishing and promoting community relationships is not a solo responsibility: it is a shared responsibility of the board, medical staff, administration, and every employee. Community partnerships can reap solid rewards for MCH. For example, MCH's geographical area is seen as a recruiting obstacle because it is in an urban neighborhood with a perceived high crime rate. Although the statistics do not prove this, the perceptions of nurses must change in order to successfully retain and recruit staff. Jane dismissed these perceptions because they were not supported by objective data, but if the perceptions are to change, listening to the nurses' concerns, recognizing their issues, and working together to resolve the problem will be absolutely necessary for progress in retention and recruitment. The nurses' perception, real or not, of their "vulnerability to crime" must be dealt with head-on. Bringing in law enforcement and community representatives to meet with the nursing leadership and hospital staff to examine factual data and to develop a system of security measures (such as escorts, community patrols, etc.) would provide concrete actions to dispel misconceptions and would help to create community partnerships.

Inviting community groups to the hospital and touring the facility is another action step to develop community coalitions. Employees and physicians meeting with community groups to talk about the hospital and its services is a useful strategy. Developing a community needs assessment to determine what services MCH should provide is a requirement and a responsibility of the board, medical staff, and administration. This assessment could be reviewed in meetings with the various groups. Contingent upon the results, services can be developed and educational sessions provided to reach out to the community and to demonstrate commitment, collaboration, and partnership.

Effective leadership is essential for MCH's survival. If the board and its chairman, senior management, and the medical staff are functioning as knowledgeable and skilled leaders, they can face the difficult problems, find solutions, and avoid problems in the future. They must be committed to the mission, vision, and values of MCH; not be afraid to face tough challenges; be willing to take risks; and be dedicated to resolving issues. Their focus must be on patient care and services, a positive organizational culture that respects employees and recognizes their value to the organization, retention and recruitment of employees and physicians, quality improvement, operational performance, and the strategic direction of the organization.

The problems and challenges at MCH are not insurmountable, but they do require concurrent efforts and strategies for resolution. If MCH is to survive and thrive in a tougher healthcare environment, all constituencies must feel engaged in the transition and participate in decision-making, and they must be valued for their input and recognized for their work. Everyone in the organization must understand the mission, vision, values, and the strategic framework and direction and believe that they can *support and promote* the actions being implemented at MCH. A unifying force of effective leadership is needed to transform the organization into one of compassion, integrity, and respect; high-quality patient care and services; and a magnet for recruiting and retaining staff and physicians.

REFERENCES

Bader, B. S. and S. O'Malley, 2000. "Putting all the pieces together: The complete board needs the right mix of competences." *Trustee* **53**(3)

Collins, J., 2001. *Good To Great*. New York: HarperCollins.

Orlikoff, J. and M. Totten, 2000. "Stewardship for the future." *Trustee* **53(1)**

Quinn, J. F., 2002. "Revisioning the nurse shortage: a call to caring for healing the healthcare system." *Frontiers of Health Services Management* **19(2)**

Romano, M., 2002. "A strong attraction." *Modern Healthcare* **32(50)**

Smith, A. P., 2002. "Evidence of our instincts: an interview with Linda H. Aiken." *Nursing Economics* **20(2)**.

The Founders Council Executive Summary, 2000. *Best Practices In Retention.* Washington, DC: The Advisory Board Company

Tyler, J. L. and E. Biggs, 2001. *Practical Governance.* Chicago: Health Administration Press

Wolf, E. J., 2001. "Four strategies for successful recruitment and retention." *Healthcare Executive* **16(4)**

9

Information technology setback: Heartland Healthcare System

Jack Moore had been frustrated throughout most of his career. Information technology (IT) was breaking new ground throughout the medical and corporate worlds; however, Jack found himself continually compromised by unimaginative bosses and organizations crippled by a lack of resources. But it looked like things were about to change. Jack had been recently hired as the chief information officer (CIO) of Heartland Healthcare System (HHS), a successful multi-hospital system. It was his dream position.

The flagship 500-bed hospital was located in the major metropolitan area of a pre-dominantly rural state in the Great Plains region. HHS's five smaller hospitals of fifty beds or fewer were scattered throughout the rural regions of the state within a 100-mile radius of Heartland. In addition, three specialty hospitals (Heart, Pediatrics, and Orthopedics) thrived in the metropolitan area along with a very busy outpatient surgi-center. The hospitals comprising HHS were connected by a sophisticated helicopter transport system that quickly transported patients in need to the flagship hospital. The hospital system employed over 5,000 staff members and 300 physicians, mostly sub-specialists. An additional 900 private practice physicians had privileges at HHS. Heartland's staff included a sizeable number of nurse practitioners who played a significant role in the care of the state's rural population and who also staffed a number of the primary healthcare clinics located in the metropolitan area.

In 1999, when Jack was hired as CIO at Heartland, he was charged with two major responsibilities: (1) To assure access and interconnectivity of medical information among all of the system's hospitals, urgent care centers, primary care clinics, and private physician offices; (2) Make HHS Y2K compliant. To make his job easier, he would report directly to the CEO.

Richard Smith had been the CEO of HHS for over fifteen years and was largely respon-sible for the success of the system. His one disappointment had been his inability to enhance the IT at Heartland. His failure to do so was in some measure attributable to John Forbes, the previous CIO who was retiring after over twenty years with Heartland and who

Management Mistakes in Healthcare, ed. Paul Hofmann and Frankie Perry. Published by Cambridge University Press. © Cambridge University Press 2005.

was thought to be out-of-date with the current available technology. Truth to tell, Richard had often berated himself for not investing more in IT and for not forcing early retirement upon John in order to better achieve this goal.

Richard was pleased with his recruitment of Jack who had very impressive IT credentials, although not in healthcare, and seemed competent and eager to move Heartland into the next generation of IT. Richard assured Jack that the needed resources had been budgeted and approved to achieve rapid progress, based upon an earlier feasibility study by a reputable IT consulting firm. The firm had been engaged to conduct the study, and both Richard and the Heartland board had been pleased with the firm's work. The IT consultants had indicated in their study that the existing CMS system at Heartland could be upgraded to make it Y2K compliant for a cost of $3 million. This seemed like a reasonable solution to the immediate problem, but Jack felt it was a myopic strategy if Heartland were to move into future cutting-edge technologies necessary to maintain its command of the market. And it certainly did not mesh with his personal ambition to build an IT system at Heartland that would be the envy of healthcare organizations across the Midwest. Given Richard's enthusiasm to bring Heartland's system up-to-date as quickly as possible, it did not take much to convince Richard of the wisdom inherent in Jack's strategy. Subsequently, a three-vendor search and a formal bid process yielded a $10 million contract with MedCor to implement a new IT system with promises of Y2K compliance and the desired interconnectivity throughout HHS.

As the project progressed, Jack hired Les Atkins, a local independent contractor, to manage the hardware conversion. This was a much more complex undertaking than Jack's previous experience had prepared him for but he felt that with Les to help him, the project would move forward. As work progressed, Jack found himself relying increasingly on Les and his advice on managing the project. Les began contracting for more and more staff time from his firm to work on the implementation, even though using Heartland IT staff would have been less expensive and certainly better for Heartland staff morale. The IT staff were beginning to grumble that they were being left out of the loop and did not know what was going on. This sense of being "left out" of the decision-making on the implementation began to escalate as the accounting staff responsible for patient billing and the nursing staff responsible for patient care were ignored. The nursing staff became especially vocal in their chagrin at not being consulted as decisions were made that impacted their patient care activities. The Vice President for Nursing wasted no time in making her concerns known to the CEO, but they were largely ignored. Richard thought this was yet another example of her marginal cooperation with other departments throughout the organization, a problem he had raised previously during her last annual performance review.

To the hospital staff, it seemed that the CIO and the manager for hardware conversion were making decisions in isolation and had the unflinching support of the CEO. To the CEO, it seemed that the hospital staff, especially Nursing, was typically being resistant to change and attempting to thwart the forward progress necessary to bring Heartland into twenty-first-century IT.

As staff morale plummeted, speculation among the staff began to focus on the appropriateness of Les' firm's business transactions with Heartland. The Purchasing staff let it be known that the acquisition of some forty keyboards and mice were purchased from Les' firm by Heartland without a formal bid process.

Then the unthinkable happened. Two years into the contract and $8 million into the $10 million project, MedCor was sold to another company and the patient accounting/billing system product that was an integral part of the Heartland project was dropped by the company. Nothing in the contract protected Heartland from this occurrence. In an effort to minimize the financial loss, Jack went back to CMS, who said with the remaining budget of $2 million, they could make Heartland Y2K compliant.

Richard was dumbfounded. Jack had recommended MedCor so strongly and was so confident that it was the perfect fit for Heartland. Following the initial shock of the disclosure however, Jack was able to convince Richard that there was no way that this unfortunate turn of events could have been foreseen. In his words, "it was a minor setback that would not prevent Heartland from moving into the technology future they both desired." In the aftermath of the MedCor débâcle, Les was hired by Heartland as its full-time Manager of Hardware Support. Jack was shaken by the MedCor departure and believed that he needed Les even more. It was common knowledge among the Heartland IT staff that Les had no formal degree; not only were the requirements for the position waived, it was also noted by the staff that no posting for the position had occurred.

Richard still has high hopes that Heartland can achieve state-of-the-art technology emulated after hardware system giants in the corporate world. While he has less confidence in Jack, and he suspects that Jack is more interested in building his own personal technology empire, he does not necessarily see their goals as being mutually exclusive. The hospital IT staff clearly lacks confidence in Jack's leadership ability. They see a firewall between the employees doing application support and IT management. The nursing staff believe that Jack has no concept of the hospital's mission as patient care and no interest in involving patient care staff in technology planning and implementation. The accounting staff are convinced that Jack has no business savvy and does not adequately focus on business applications. In fact, one employee was recently overheard to say, "Jack is more intent on being a cutting-edge IT think tank than being an integral part of a hospital system whose job is to serve patients."

Commentary

Mark R. Neaman

HHS and its CEO, Richard Smith, have much to celebrate. A progressive clinical enterprise, with substantial growth and geographic reach, the system is the envy of many. Richard, as the chief architect of the system development these past fifteen years, should take pride in these achievements, as well as being able to survive the "wars" for such a substantial period of time.

So what is the issue at Heartland? Perhaps, one word summarizes the issue – "frustration." This case of IT gone awry is a classic situation of a high-tech failure with compounded consequences for individuals and organizations alike. Who has not been frustrated or disappointed with the results of major IT decisions? The scope of IT's frustrating failure at Heartland, however, goes well beyond economic considerations, and underscores a much more significant "crisis of confidence" in the very leadership capabilities of those at the top.

There are many lessons here to be learned (or re-learned) from the case study at HHS. An unbundling of some of the myriad factors leading to the crisis now evident should prove useful in shedding some light on at least a few of the mistakes along the way.

Richard Smith, by virtue of his position as CEO, naturally, gets a disproportionate share of the blame for the circumstances surrounding this case. The first contributing factor is a *failure of strategy* (not technology). Richard's strategy, fermented in frustration, seems to be one of making more IT investments, no matter the cost or value. Further, this strategy is divorced from the traditional elements of a solid overall, corporate-wide strategy, including such imperatives as growth, low-cost relative position, or market share leader. In fact, the IT strategy is not a strategy at all – but simply some confusing tactics to have HHS become a great IT shop, not necessarily a great healthcare institution. The divorcing of the IT tactics strategy from the corporate strategy is then fatally compounded by the separation of IT from operations. Who is the champion of the cause from the operations staff? Even the most brilliant strategies fail due to the fact that only empowered operations leaders can *implement* the strategy and really make it work. It is at best an illusion to believe success is achievable without flawless execution.

Fifteen contributing factors to this IT crisis are:

 (1) A failure of *strategy* (not technology)
 (2) The *divorcing* of *strategy*, *tactics*, and *operations* from each other
 (3) An absence of *goals and measures of success*
 (4) A failure to diagnose *underlying organizational psychology*
 (5) A failure to hire the *right people*
 (6) A failure to distinguish between *means* and *ends*
 (7) An absence of *support and accountability*
 (8) The *ill-defined role of consultants* and *outsourcing* arrangements
 (9) A breakdown in adhering to *purchasing protocols*
(10) A failure to prevent *intra-staff* "warfare"
(11) The lack of "openness" in *contracting*
(12) A failure to confront the *allegations of impropriety*

(13) A failure to *learn from other industries*

(14) A failure to function as an *integrated team*

(15) A failure to fire *Jack Moore.*

The only strategy that appears to be set by either CEO Smith or CIO Moore are some very loose and mystical goals, such as "interconnectivity" and "award winning." For a $10 million investment, the CEO must establish *institutional clarity* for outcomes and appropriate signposts and measures of success along the way. Non-specific, illusive goals like "improved interconnectivity" could be achieved simply by adding more telephones – or if you really want to be high-tech, wireless telephones! The CEO's expressed goal of "enhancing IT," along with Jack Moore's ambition to build an IT system that "would be the envy of healthcare organizations across the Midwest," is egocentric, not value-centric. If these are the real intended goals, at least set up a measure of success for the number of external awards won.

Perhaps part of the underlying cause for the elusiveness of specific goals and measures for the Heartland system is the lack of a *truly integrated enterprise*. Other than the helicopter service (flying between the main hospital and its satellites), is this really a fully integrated system, or simply a series of parts? Are the 300 physicians in the practice group fully integrated and practicing as a Mayo Clinic-type group? Are the 5,000 staff members all on the same payroll, purchasing, and financial systems or separate at each hospital campus? The stated goal of improved interconnectivity suggests that many of these basic system integrators are either not in place, or are weak. Nevertheless, the failure to establish *explicit goals with defined measures of success* is a significant contributor to the demise of this or any major IT project. To overcome this failure, specific goals – such as reducing the number of medical errors, driving down costs per case, improving turnaround time for results, or improving service to increase the number of referrals – are all examples of appropriate goals and measures of success for this type of project.

A fourth contributing factor at HHS lies in a failure to understand *organizational psychology and people*. CEO Smith has fallen into the trap of symbolism over substance. Having the new CIO Moore report directly to the CEO in order to make his job easier is a classic mistake. Smith's institutional message in having Moore directly report to him is really nothing more than a veiled threat to the organization that "you better make this work because the new guy is reporting to me." It also assures that others on the management team will either be envious of Moore's reporting relationship or washing their hands of any IT projects as "not my job." Every support department probably wants to report to the CEO for increased visibility and the likely additional resources that might come their way through this reporting relationship. Heartland is big enough, however, to have IT report to its COO or similar role in the corporate offices. Keep in mind, as well, that Heartland is a healthcare organization and not an IT corporation. The organizational alignments must be centered on the efficient delivery of healthcare services with areas like IT playing a *supportive* role, not the lead role.

In additional to the misdiagnosed organizational psychology, Jack Moore was simply a bad hire for the CIO position. Moore is competent, with a good technological background and successes in other industries. The fact that he has grown up in non-healthcare industries is not the issue; the issue is his focus on "personal ambition," rather than system success and his lack of interpersonal leadership skills. Moore admits to continuously being frustrated by unimaginative bosses and lack of resources. Each of his previous bosses have likely been significantly burned by past failures in IT and a natural reticence to throw more resources on top of past failures. Moore's personality type of "no patience, blames others, not a team player," and personal ambition, is a surefire formula for failure. The IT staff deservedly lacks confidence in his leadership ability, and got it exactly right when they noted he is "more intent on being a cutting edge IT think tank than being an integral part of a hospital system, whose job is to serve patients." Moore is technically competent, but technical competence is not nearly enough – *leadership and people skills* remain pre-eminent requisites for any successful endeavor.

The mistakes associated with organizational psychology and people leads naturally into a sixth area of misstep, namely the confusion of *means* and *ends*. This is a major responsibility of any good CEO. The effective CEO must be able to design and communicate a specific vision for the organization at least three–five years into the future. This is the endpoint. The means for achieving that vision typically require multiple tactics and measures along the way to assure you are on the right road in achieving that vision. Achieving HHS's vision of being a strong, growing, clinically excellent healthcare enterprise will require multiple inputs, and IT will be one of the important tools to accomplish this end. What needs to occur is to de-couple the notion that IT's interconnectivity is the end point – it is merely one of the means to help achieve that vision.

A seventh clear organizational failure is the lack of building even a modest basis of *support and accountability* for successful implementation of the IT systems. Some may argue that what is required is 100% participation and buy in by all parties to such situations before moving ahead. If that were true, nothing would ever happen and the CEO's frustration level would be incalculable. What is needed organizationally is to place the accountability for designing and measuring the desired outcomes for the IT systems in the hands of one or more of the operating VPs. Establishing this accountability – with appropriate measures and rewards – will do more to assure a favorable outcome of the project than almost any other single factor. Operational accountability, by its very nature, will also assure the building of bridges to other areas of the operation along with a requirement for strong IT staff support. There is currently no accountability with operations at HHS for this project. Even if CIO Moore were to somehow implement the software, would anyone care?

An eighth contributing factor in the IT crisis at HHS is the ill-defined role of *consultants and outsourcing arrangements* that have percolated through the IT ranks. The only thing worse for the psyche of an organization than hiring a consultant is to hire a consultant and then fully ignore her advice; this is exactly what HHS has done. This leads to (a) significant insecurity as to what direction the organization is taking and (b) legitimate complaints from employees that the institution wastes substantial amounts of money on outsiders that could more appropriately be in their paychecks. The IT consultant identified an immediate and critical requirement that systems be Y2K compliant; failure to do so would shut down the entire enterprise. Dismissing this as a "myopic strategy" is at best disingenuous, if not injurious to the corporation. Perhaps, the best solution to the Y2K issue was indeed the decision to go with the major overhaul with MedCor. To ignore the Y2K landmine identified by the external consultant was not a trivial matter.

Jack shows his maverick style in the decisions both to outsource to Les Atkins the hardware conversion and the $10 million contract with MedCor. Outsourcing, in and of itself, is not the issue; outsourcing is frequently a superior approach to a given operation than trying to do it oneself. This is particularly true in cases like HHS where recruiting specific expertise may be difficult, when the scope is beyond one's reasonable core capabilities, or where the project is time-limited. It would appear that Jack performed little due diligence on Les and made no provision for a "backup" for him, thus becoming more and more dependent upon him as a contractor. With no other choices available, HHS finds itself now in a *de facto* long-term outsourced agreement that the leadership never really anticipated or announced to the organization. The lack of clear boundaries and accountabilities for the outsourced contractor predictably created much grumbling among the Heartland staff and left them out of the decision-making process. One can imagine further that the IT staff is also looking over their shoulders to see if their jobs will be similarly outsourced in the near future. Les' firm appears to be technically competent and is apparently filling the void created by Jack Moore's absence during the implementation process. Backing into this outsourcing arrangement, however, looks, feels, and is deceptive. Successful outsourcing agreements must overcome a natural *credibility and threat gap*, as well as the relationship gap that naturally exists between in-house and outsourced services.

An interesting and important irritant that has come from Moore's mismanagement of the outsourcing relationship is with the VP for Nursing. The frustration of the VP for Nursing in not being apprised of major decisions that affect her operating responsibilities is escalating. She approaches the CEO – Jack Moore's boss – with these concerns. Why not approach Jack Moore? This is another reason why the CIO should not be reporting to Richard Smith. There is now no room for compromise; it's winner take all in the game of whom the CEO will support. Richard doesn't have time for this animosity and lack of cooperation; you can hear him say: "there goes Nursing – totally uncooperative as usual." This is obviously not a new issue in the relationship between nursing, Richard, and the other senior managers. Richard may soon be berating himself for not forcing early retirement upon the VP of Nursing, just like he did with the previous CIO, John Forbes. Remember, the nurses at HHS are truly the key care-givers and the true inter-connectivity in the system today. There is much to lose here in the *very core of the HHS care mission* if Nursing now goes awry.

A further failure of HHS, which contributes substantially to the current IT crisis, is the complete breakdown in adherence to *purchasing protocols*. The implementation of the MedCor contact appears to be a unilateral decision by the maverick CIO. Purchasing clearly has been left out of the process, and Finance's only involvement seems to be to pay the bills. With the benefit of hindsight, we see that Jack has opened HHS to charges of impropriety, as well as the loss of substantial economic resources.

Heartland did the right thing in at least going through the process of a vendor search and formal bid process leading to the selection of MedCor. From there, who negotiated and executed the contract? It appears that Jack took care of this himself without sign-off by the purchasing department or legal counsel. Any basic contract for software from a vendor such as MedCor would have guarantees that, should the company go out of business, be acquired, or discontinue the product, at least the software code would be made available to HHS. Having bypassed these standard purchasing guarantees and relying simply on the bid process, Jack has caused HHS an $8 million loss with nothing to show for it now that MedCor is out of business.

Knowing that purchasing protocols were disregarded, the purchasing staff will not be hesitant in bringing attention to Jack's errors. It doesn't take long. The sweetheart deal between Jack and Les Atkins creates tremendous vulnerability for the organization. As soon as the forty keyboards come up missing, the purchasing staff quickly "blows the whistle." In an era where corporate compliance and integrity in all aspects of business, but certainly in purchasing and contracts, is essential, this failure is indefensible. Protocols, including purchasing procedures, have a purpose. They provide essential checks and balances in the system to help assure that multiple parties look at the proposed acquisition from a variety of perspectives. Complying with good protocols can minimize the possibility of problems, or at least provide some early warning signs of likely trouble in the future. Whether Jack and outsource contractor Les are really in a nefarious relationship is unknown; I frankly doubt it. Regardless of fact, the whole organization believes there is something wrong here and the perception has become the reality. All of this would have been prevented by following HHS's standard acquisition and contracting guidelines at the outset.

Richard Smith and the leadership at Heartland have missed an opportunity (as opposed to making a mistake) related to the system's selection of Jack Moore. He is "a distinguished IT executive" with experience from other industries. How has HHS benefited from his broad perspective? Assuming that interconnectivity was the right goal and clearly defined, what have other industries learned in addressing this question? For example, airlines, banking and retailing all face similar questions, given multiple transactions and multiple sites in their system requirements.

One has to wonder if Jack has seen the successful deployment of such systems in the non-healthcare organizations where he has already provided leadership. If HHS were to address the question of interconnectivity not simply as a medical issue, but as a "business issue," the universe of appropriate supporting companies, software systems, and alternatives would have exponentially increased to HSS. Perhaps this would have even precluded the crisis fueled by the fall of MedCor. It is unfortunate that Richard states his dream to achieve state-of-the-art technology based upon the "system giants in the corporate world," while apparently ignoring the experience of these giants.

Jack Moore has an unhealthy hold on his CEO. Stemming from Richard Smith's failure to organize properly, his only IT resource is his CIO, all other voices are "uncooperative" – or, worse, silent. On occasion, the CEO's role, by virtue of its position within the organizational hierarchy, can become isolated. The CEO must work hard at developing multiple trusted IT resources, including those not depicted on the organization chart. It is healthy and worthwhile, not counter-productive, to have multiple perspectives: sometimes, they even agree. The "silo mentality" at HHS that seems to characterize the CEO, CIO, Accounting, Purchasing, Nursing, and the rest, raises the question: do they ever even meet together as a group? Smith must find ways to promote *interdisciplinary actions and accountability* across his wide system. Giving direct assignments to his key staff beyond their immediate "four walls" will require everyone to talk with one another and be mutually accountable. Underscoring these joint responsibilities with *mutual incentive compensation goals* would also do much for collaboration at HHS.

The final evidence of Jack Moore's unhealthy hold on his CEO is when the MedCor system collapses. Jack's reaction was: "It was a minor setback." Richard should be outraged. Jack's decision has cost HHS not only $8 million dollars in capital, but fueled significant animosity among the staff, and questioned the very integrity of the people and systems at HHS essential to the core functioning of the organization. Jack's employment must be terminated.

The crisis of confidence associated with the IT miscues clearly has many contributing factors. No attempt has been made to list each and every contributing factor, particularly those that are self-evident, or need no further comment. Obvious abuses, such as violating the company's hiring practices in the employment of Les Atkins or the destructive "firewall" between IT management and the applications support personnel are issues, but are more the products of other underlying causes. A final aspect of the case, however, which is not typical, relates to *resource allocation*. IT investments frequently do suffer from underfunding. This is not the case at HHS, where more than sufficient financial resources, particularly in support of hardware and software, had been made available. The CEO made it clear – this project will not fail from a lack of resources. The ultimate management mistake at HHS was the failure to recognize that financial resources, regardless of quantity, are never sufficient in and of themselves. Acquiring even the very best of hardware and software without sufficient training and testing of empowered people employed to utilize the system will invariably come up short.

Richard Smith is an accomplished and long-tenured CEO. He can overcome the significant failures and mistakes associated with the most recent MedCor IT system decisions and related events. To do so, he must move quickly to restore the confidence and trust in himself and those who are leading the organization.

10

Inept strategic planning: Southwestern Regional Healthcare System

Southwestern Regional Healthcare System (SRHS) is a highly respected regional referral system located in a major metropolitan area of the Southwest. Its 800-bed Medical Center houses a number of tertiary care programs equipped with the latest technology and staffed by highly competent specialist and subspecialist physicians and well-trained nurses. Its Level 1 Trauma Center is supported by a Surgical ICU, a Pediatric ICU, a Neonatal ICU, a Burn Center, and a Cardiac ICU. In addition, the system operates an emergency medical transport program that includes helicopters to bring patients in need from all regions of the state to SRHS which serves as the regional referral center for a population of just over a million.

SRHS is considered the marquee hospital within its metropolitan area where University Hospital, St. Anne's, and HSA, a for-profit hospital, are also located. In addition to its critical care capabilities and its general medical–surgical programs, SRHS has committed considerable resources to its obstetrics program in an attempt to increase its dwindling market share within the community.

SRHS' Board of Governors, medical staff leadership, and management staff recently convened for a major strategic planning retreat during which its obstetrics program received considerable attention. Increasing the obstetrical patient volume, specifically normal deliveries, was a focus of discussion. Strategies for achieving this goal centered on capturing the rising OB market of LaPaz, a border town some 100 miles south of SRHS. A high-tech manufacturing firm had recently relocated one of its plants to this small town and its economy, as well as its population, was on the rise. The healthcare capabilities within this rapidly growing town of 35,000 residents were being strained. It had been difficult attracting physicians to this small, previously rural community, and a primary care group practice of three physicians provided the majority of care for the town's residents. A small, twenty-bed hospital provided emergency care and hospitalization for patients who could be cared for there. Others drove or were transported to the cities to the north or

Management Mistakes in Healthcare, ed. Paul Hofmann and Frankie Perry. Published by Cambridge University Press. © Cambridge University Press 2005.

west of LaPaz. The rapidly increasing population of LaPaz consisted mostly of young, family-oriented couples eager to settle down within this promising community.

The decision-makers at SRHS believed that the situation was ideal for a satellite OB hospital where SRHS obstetricians could perform normal deliveries and helicopter high-risk patients back to the flagship hospital. This strategy could increase the SRHS OB patient volume in both normal deliveries and high-risk cases. SRHS had the resources, the prestige, and the "brand" name recognition that would most certainly be attractive to patients. And, given the current situation, it would be the only game in town. The board appointed a subcommittee to investigate the availability and costs of appropriate proper-ties upon which to build a satellite OB facility in LaPaz. Administration was directed to put together a business plan for the project, including how the new satellite facility would be promoted within the community.

The SRHS OB satellite opened ten months later with much celebration and optimism, but its promising future never came to fruition. While there were many normal deliveries occurring within the LaPaz community, very few of them were taking place at the SRHS satellite facility. The young pregnant women in LaPaz continued to go to the primary group practice for their pre-natal care and continued to have their deliveries performed by these family doctors or in their private homes by midwives, which had been the prevailing custom. The women in LaPaz had been comfortable with these care-givers in the past and saw no reason to change now. The primary care group practice snubbed the SRHS obstetricians entirely and continued to send their high-risk patients to the city west of LaPaz. It was clear they resented what they viewed as a "hostile takeover attempt" by SRHS and, while they were cordial, they directed their referrals elsewhere.

SRHS administrators met with the single major employer in LaPaz in an attempt to negotiate a preferred provider agreement, but the manufacturing firm declined and continued to offer its employees indemnity insurance coverage that it believed to be less expensive and less hassle than SRHS services. As they explained it, their employees were very happy with their existing healthcare coverage and related services, and they liked the choices available to them.

Commentary

Robert S. Bonney

Overview: a taste of organizational arrogance

This case presents several interesting issues which all seem to center around the key principle that was forgotten: *every market is different*, and what works in one market may not work in another.

SRHS approached the planning for this new hospital, as it would have for a service located in its market, a major metropolitan area of the Southwest, rather than a small rural border community 100 miles from a major metropolitan area.

SRHS is considered the marquee hospital within its metropolitan area. With marquee status often comes a bit of organizational arrogance and an attitude that the organization knows what is best. Organizations with this kind of market presence need to guard against this, but SRHS appears to have fallen into this trap. According to the case, "SRHS had the resources, the prestige, and the 'brand' name recognition that would most certainly be attractive to patients." They assumed their marquee status would follow them to LaPaz and that everyone would welcome the opportunity to have their babies delivered at their OB hospital; after all, they were the best. They forgot to ask their future customers what they wanted.

Business planning process

The case study implies that little real *business planning* was done, other than a review of the demographics and a development of the financial projections. The demographic analysis led to the creation of a financial plan, based on assumptions about the community and likely use of the proposed facility, which showed that the project was feasible. The key to any business plan is the *assumptions*. It is important to confirm the assumptions that are made to the best of your ability. It is obvious that little effort was made to confirm the many assumptions that went into the financial plan.

A comprehensive business plan would have also included, among other things:
- An analysis of the *needs and wants* of the population
- A review of existing area physicians' and other providers' *practices and referral patterns*
- A review of the *employers' and payers'* views of the project
- The plan to *promote the facility* in the community
- Influence of the *existing hospital* on the primary care physicians
- The *governance structure* of the facility.

An analysis of the needs and wants of the population

In addition to reviewing the demographic data, it is important to understand how healthcare is delivered in a community, and the needs and wants of that community. Often what is wanted is not necessarily needed, and what objectively can be determined to be needed is not wanted. For example, women want to stay in the hospital for two days following a normal delivery and four days following a cesarean section but there is no objective data showing that patients (either moms or babies) have better outcomes than those who stay a shorter time in the hospital and have home care follow up. Thus, what is wanted by the patient is different from what is objectively needed. In this case, women appear to be satisfied with the care they are receiving and thus the need for a higher quality of obstetrical care does not match the want.

A valuable tool in developing a business plan is surveying the community to determine its members' needs and wants. This may be done by mail, personal interviews, or even focus groups. Such a survey could have been used to ascertain:
- If the "marquee status" of SRHS *really existed* in LaPaz
- If the community identified a *need* for better OB services and whether or not they would use these services if SRHS brought new services to town
- The use by the community of *midwives*
- The community's view of the *quality of care* of the existing providers, both physicians and midwives
- What the community felt would be important to make an OB hospital *successful* in the market
- Key elements necessary to *promote the new hospital* in the community.

Had a survey been conducted, SRHS would have had a better understanding of the community and would have been able to develop an *implementation plan* designed to meet its needs. Further, the assumptions that were made in the business and financial plan would have been tested, thereby making them more reliable. Finally, SRHS would have been better able to position itself to develop community support for the project before it began the construction.

A review of existing area physicians' and other providers' practices and referral patterns

SRHS forgot that the number one way people select a provider of healthcare is by asking their friends, neighbors, or their primary care physician. Understanding the community's feeling toward the existing providers would have aided SRHS in positioning their OB physicians. SRHS assumed that the population of LaPaz would want care delivered by OB physicians, since this is what the metropolitan community they currently served wanted. In addition, the medical community of SRHS believed that OB physicians provided the best quality of obstetric care.

As was pointed out in the case, the referral of complex cases is currently going to the north and west of LaPaz. No attempt was made to determine why these patterns existed. It could have been that these physicians trained in the community to which they were referring, and they were well known to the referring LaPaz physicians. It could have been that they also traveled to LaPaz a couple of times a year to conduct continuing education programs for the LaPaz physicians. Maybe some of these physicians invited the LaPaz physicians on hunting and fishing trips with them at their cabins. Whatever the reason, their relationships with those referring physicians had been long-standing. If they were getting good service from these physicians and were satisfied with the quality of care received by their patients, SRHS should have realized that it would be hard to redirect these referrals. The physicians from SRHS would be seen as outsiders, trying to get the benefits of the growth that was occurring in town, where previously they had not paid any attention to LaPaz.

SRHS should have determined what motivated the local physicians to send their current referrals away from them to other communities. SRHS should have determined what needs the local providers had that were not being met by those currently getting the referrals. As part of the business planning process, SRHS should have determined what it would take to redirect these referrals. If this redirection were unlikely to occur, then a strategy needed to be developed on how to appeal to the local public and bypass the primary care physicians.

In addition, the use of midwives should have been explored further. The local community was satisfied using midwives and the midwives had apparently carved out a niche for themselves that met their patients' needs as well as the needs of the local primary care physicians. Local customs and practices encouraged the use of midwives. Perhaps SRHS should have attempted to develop a model that incorporated these midwives in the planning and operation of the new hospital, even to the point of employing them on the staff.

It is obvious that by not including the local providers in the planning and development of the new hospital, SRHS made a serious mistake. They assumed that they would be welcomed into the community as there was a need for better obstetrical care. By involving the local providers, SRHS would have learned their concerns and been in a better position to anticipate the eventual outcome and to plan for it. They might have been able to get the existing medical group's support in a variety of ways. For example, since the group was having problems recruiting physicians to the area, they could have worked out recruitment support for a family practice physician who also did obstetrical care to join the group. By helping the group meet the needs of the growing community by adding to their group, and protecting the group's income both from the start-up costs associated with a new physician and from potential competition from other primary care physicians in the process, SRHS might have been able to garner the support of the primary care physicians. This, however, would mean that SRHS would likely have had to compromise its view regarding the delivery of obstetrical care (which this author assumes relied on board-certified obstetrical physicians).

A review of the employers' and payers' views of the project

There is one major employer in LaPaz. SRHS administrators met with that employer in an attempt to negotiate a preferred provider agreement, but the manufacturing firm declined and continued to offer its employees the indemnity insurance coverage that it believed to be less expensive and less difficult to administer than SRHS services. As they explained it, their employees were very happy with their existing healthcare coverage and related services, and they liked the choices available to them.

SRHS should have been cultivating the employer and payer communities prior to initiating this project. Support from the major employer appeared to be critical because this employer was the one responsible for the growth in the community and for bringing the young families to town. By attempting to negotiate a preferred provider arrangement, SRHS was confirming what the local community already suspected – SRHS's intent was to use LaPaz for its own gain, likely at the expense of the local providers.

Since the major employer wanted to offer choice to their employees, perhaps SRHS should have just tried to get a contract with the employer and not try to get a preferred arrangement. If they were as good as they believed, they should have been able to attract patients to their hospital if given an equal chance with the other local providers. Eventually the major employer would become concerned about cost, and might then have been more agreeable to a preferred arrangement. SRHS should have identified all of the major insurance payers in the LaPaz market and should have gotten contracts to provide services for their members prior to constructing the hospital.

Influence of the existing hospital

The influence of the existing hospital should also not have been overlooked. Although it was a small hospital, it was the only hospital in the market area. It served the needs of the local physicians. Often the local hospital is the major employer in a small town; likely it was the second largest employer in this community, given that the new manufacturing firm was now there and had become the major employer in the area.

The Board of Directors of a local hospital is usually composed of key community leaders. Nothing is mentioned in the case about the board's structure at the new SRHS OB hospital, so it can be inferred that the board is from out of town. One of the strategies that SRHS should have used was to create a local Board of Directors at the inception of the project. It should have included community leaders, midwives, and physicians. These community leaders would have become vested in the project as it was being developed and would have been able to assist in the business planning for the new project, advising where there might be pitfalls to overcome.

SRHS might have found it necessary to joint venture (JV) the new hospital with the local hospital in order to get community support. Certainly there needed to be a strong working relationship with the local hospital. SRHS could have worked out arrangements whereby the local hospital provided support and services where it could, thereby neither duplicating nor competing with the local hospital.

The plan to promote the facility in the community

It appears that SRHS' plan to promote the facility was a "build it and they will come" approach. Once again, this demonstrates the organizational arrogance of SRHS. It is a highly respected regional referral system in a major metropolitan area, and its leaders know what is best. However, they do not understand the LaPaz community. They apparently believed that all they needed to do was let the local community know they were ready to serve them and they would come.

If SRHS' plan was not to involve the local community providers and leaders in the planning and development of the new OB hospital, then it needed a plan to *market directly* to the local population. Assuming it had contracts with the payers that offer insurance in LaPaz – a critical assumption – then they needed to develop a direct-to-consumer marketing approach. Such a direct-to-consumer approach would be a high-risk one aimed at pointing out why SRHS' facility provided the best care in town, or the risks to their unborn infants women faced by not using the facility. Emphasis would be on the risks associated with using other limited-access facilities, or the dangers of traveling too far, or other fear-raising concerns. By employing such a strategy, SRHS would be implying that the local providers were inferior to SRHS, and could alienate the local providers for a long time to come.

Summary

This case illustrates what can happen when a premier healthcare institution relies on its "marquee status" in one market to penetrate a market in a different geographical area. As noted previously, the behavior exhibited by SRHS was *organizational arrogance*, conveying an attitude of "what is good for SRHS is good for LaPaz." SRHS forgot that every market is different, and that what works in one market may not work in another market.

SRHS should have developed "buy in" for their project by involving the local community providers and leaders in the planning and development of the project. If these people resisted, at least SRHS would have known what it was up against. It needed to confirm its assumptions regarding the market's needs and wants: at the very least, involving or attempting to involve these parties would have done that. SRHS could have then structured a plan to address these concerns and foster acceptance of their project.

SRHS needed to realize that a business plan is not just a financial plan, which is all they had. The business plan should have included, as a minimum:

- An analysis of the needs and wants of the population
- A review of existing area physicians' and other providers' practices and referral patterns
- A review of the employers' and payers' views of the project
- The plan to promote the facility in the community, including a strategy for getting support of the project from the local business leaders
- The influence of the existing hospital
- The governance structure of the facility.

A plan is as good only as the assumptions upon which it is based, and confirmation of these assumptions is critical to success.

In summary, SRHS made numerous mistakes in their planning for this project; chief among them was assuming that the LaPaz market would respond as the SRHS market would, without testing this assumption. This basic assumption was the underpinning of the financial plan that led to the decision to proceed. SRHS' business planning process was flawed in that it appeared to involve only data analysis and financial projections, and did not contain a thorough analysis of the product's *acceptance in the market*. Involving – or, at least, attempting to involve – the local provider and public community in the planning and execution of this project would have given this project a better chance of success.

11

Public relations fiasco, George C. Fremont Community Hospital

The George C. Fremont Community Hospital (FCH) is located in a mid-sized West Coast city that is regarded as an attractive retirement community. It has been heavily endowed by its namesake, and its governing board and management are working diligently to compete with the more prominent healthcare facilities in the nearby larger cities. To better serve its retired community, FCH has focused on the more significant healthcare needs of its residents and has developed a state-of-the-art Cardiology program. FCH has been successful in attracting local residents in need into its program and has gained a solid reputation within the community as the desirable provider of cardiac care services.

Brad Holmes has been the CEO of FCH since it opened six years ago and is proud of the progress of the organization which he knows is the result of hard work and commitment on the part of the FCH staff. Brad was shocked and ill prepared for the report that he received from his COO, Grace Selby, this morning. With grave concern, he was told that a patient died earlier in the day during his cardiac catheterization because he received a lethal dose of nitrous oxide instead of the oxygen that should have been given. It appears that the deadly error was the result of malfunctioning equipment that was known to be defective and should have been repaired. In fact, the staff responsible for the maintenance of medical equipment was visibly shaken but could offer no excuse for overlooking this needed repair.

Brad was appalled and felt the damage to the hospital's reputation and its future could be disastrous. In a rage, he told Grace to fire those responsible and to set up a meeting immediately with the patient's physicians. In Brad's opinion, this was a crisis that had to be contained. Because he was determined to keep the details of this tragic event confidential, he vetoed Grace's suggestion that the management staff in the cardiac catheterization lab and biomedical engineering be included in the meeting. Brad asked the physicians what the patient's family had been told of the incident and the cause of death. The primary care physician reported that he had met with the family and told them that the patient had a severe adverse reaction to the anesthetic resulting in a cardiac arrest and could not be revived. He said that he honestly believed that to be the case when he met with the family. It was only subsequent to that meeting that he learned of the nitrous

Management Mistakes in Healthcare, ed. Paul Hofmann and Frankie Perry. Published by Cambridge University Press. © Cambridge University Press 2005.

oxide inhalation. Brad was visibly relieved and asked that the physicians not disclose any additional information to the family until he had a chance to assess the hospital's position and response. The physicians reluctantly agreed.

Next, Brad met with the Director of Media Relations, Jordan White. After detailing the events of the morning, Brad asked that Jordan develop a comprehensive plan with strategies designed to contain this information within the confines of those staff who currently knew the details of the incident. Brad emphasized that the cause of death must not be made public, indicating that any media inquiries were to be handled personally by Jordan and were to be treated as though this incident had not occurred. When Jordan offered advice counter to this, Brad cut him short and repeated that this incident was not to be made public at all costs. When Jordan asked if he should prepare a briefing for the board, Brad repeated that the details of the incident would remain within the confidence of those currently informed, and it was Jordan's job to assure this outcome.

Following Jordan's departure, Brad asked his administrative assistant to get the hospital's legal counsel on the line and then retreated into his office to think about how to handle the attorney who might advocate some kind of disclosure. Brad was determined not to have that happen. After all, he reflected, disclosure could serve no good purpose. It would not bring the patient back. As Brad waited for the hospital attorney to return his call, Jordan knocked on his door. He reported that when he returned to his office, there had been a phone message for him from the local newspaper inquiring about the deceased patient.

Commentary

Ruth M. Rothstein,
Chief, Cook Country Bureau of Health Services

Overview

The Board of Trustees, the CEO, and staff of FCH have made tremendous strides in meeting the needs of the hospital's community. They have spent the past six years building the hospital's reputation as having a state-of-the art Cardiology program and as "the" desirable provider of cardiac care services, albeit to attract patients in a competitive marketplace. In a mere six hours, that reputation can be irreparably harmed by the CEO's response, or lack of response, to a medical error that occurred during a routine cardiology procedure. In his zealousness to protect the institution's (and his own) reputation, the CEO takes immediate action. Unfortunately, his actions are ultimately not in the best interest of good patient care nor in the best interest of the hospital. It is the CEO's response to this error, and not the error itself, which may very well cost the hospital and himself their well-earned reputations.

Management mistakes

When the medical error was brought to the attention of Brad Holmes, his immediate response was to be concerned about the reputation of the hospital, and not the effect on the patient. He reacted by flying into a rage and, therefore, made the wrong responses. His total inclination was to keep the details of this tragic event confidential. I can understand someone initially being enraged by this situation, but this rage should have lasted for only two seconds. At this point, he should have sat down to determine the appropriate response and strategy, rather than issuing orders to fire everyone because doing so could not fix the problem. That was his first immediate error.

At this point, it seems ironic that in order to comment on management mistakes made in this case, one must make the "mistake" of assuming some facts that are not included in the synopsis and draw some conclusions that may or may not be correct. With that said, it appears that the larger mistake was made prior to this error happening. That is, hospital leadership had not clearly defined its commitment to *ensuring patient safety*. Certainly, the hospital's success in developing a state-of-the art Cardiology program demonstrated that there had been a commitment to provide excellent patient care, which in turn implies that there was an equally strong commitment towards patient safety. However, the CEO's reaction to this error demonstrates that the hospital's commitment to patient safety was not as clear as it should be.

The second error made by the CEO was his "shoot from the hip" response in wanting to keep the error a secret and not to engage in an investigative mode. His desire for secrecy is misguided and created more confusion. His vetoing the suggestion that hospital staff be included in the meeting with the physicians to discuss this case was understandable. Certainly from the perspective of possible litigation, it is obvious why he wanted to keep all information confidential and close to the vest. However, in order to get to the root of the problem and prevent it from occurring again, it is vital that the staff involved be given the opportunity to discuss and analyze this situation.

With regard to the CEO's request that the patient's physicians not disclose additional information to the patient's family until he had a chance to assess the hospital's position and response, this was an appropriate position. However, he was ignoring the fact that the physicians' concerns were that this had been a patient of theirs and they had a responsibility to inform the family of the status of the situation. The CEO should have scheduled a follow up meeting with the physicians, preferably within the hour, and also included them in further discussions.

In a case that has the potential for media coverage, the CEO's request to the Director of Media Relations to develop a strategic plan on handling information pertaining to the error was entirely appropriate. However, his desire to treat this error as though it had not occurred borders on the ridiculous. The CEO is ignoring his ethical responsibility to the patient, the medical staff, and the community with his denial and desire for absolute secrecy.

The CEO's reaction to this error appears to be the result of a failure to establish and implement: (1) an *organizational philosophy* on patient safety which includes open and honest communication between the hospital, its patients, and practitioners and (2) a defined *patient safety program* which includes systematic review, analysis, and communication of medical errors. Or, worse yet, there is the possibility that the hospital has an established philosophy and mechanisms for open communication, which the CEO has chosen to ignore. With the push towards reducing medical errors on a national basis, disclosure of problems such as this is imperative, advocated, and mandated. The CEO's efforts are counter to this. One must question the good judgment of a CEO who would keep this information from the Board of Trustees and who would underestimate the power of the media as he attempted to deny that this error occurred.

How mistakes could have been avoided

There are two categories of mistakes presented in this scenario – the mistakes that caused the patient's death and the mistakes made in responding to the death. The hospital will never get the answers to the former because of the CEO's response to this event.

Most of the management mistakes made by the CEO in this case following the discovery of the error could have been avoided if the institution had adopted an *open communication philosophy* and had adhered to the Joint Commission on Accreditation of Healthcare Organization's (JCAHO) standards on patient rights, organizational ethics, and hospital leadership's role in patient safety. The JCAHO requires that patients be informed of unanticipated outcomes and that patient safety programs address procedures for immediate response to clinical errors, mechanisms for support of staff who have been involved in a "sentinel event," a process for managing sentinel events, and clear systems for internal and external reporting of information relating to clinical errors.

That being said, even prior to the JCAHO's standards, many hospitals have successfully dealt with similar situations without elaborate plans. How? By doing the right thing ethically and by not being frozen by fear of litigation and the media.

If you were to question most professionals as to how they would respond in this situation if they knew that they would not be sued and their reputation would not be damaged, they would tell you that they would be compassionate, upfront, and honest with the patient's family about what had happened. Why? Because that is how they would want someone to treat them.

Organizational steps to prevent these mistakes in the future

The CEO, along with the Board of Trustees, must decide on what their communication philosophy is (one wonders if the CEO's communication style in this scenario was a reflection of the Board of Trustees' style). Once that is done, then clear procedures for handing medical errors must be established, consistent with the hospital's communication philosophy and JCAHO standards.

Ideally, the institution should adopt an open and honest communication style, from the Board of Trustees downward. However, as many of us know, this is easier said than done. It is not usually the "honest" communication that is difficult; it is the *openness*. Many hospitals continue to adopt a "no comment" approach to situations like this. Why? Because, allegedly, it is the safe approach. It's not being dishonest, but it certainly leaves everyone wondering whether you are hiding something, and that can be more damaging to a facility's reputation than to hit the issue straight on. Most institutions are still fumbling with being open in their communications, probably because it is a significant departure from their previous responses to situations such as this.

In our experience, we have found that in very difficult situations, the more open we have been with the patient, physicians, and leadership, the less likely it is that the media is involved. In the FCH scenario, one wonders who notified the media, and why? Was it the patient's family, or even a hospital employee, who was angry and frustrated about the information, or lack of information, that the family had been given?

As a public institution, Cook Country Hospital has certainly had its share of media attention, both positive and negative. We have avoided some negative publicity by our response to medical errors. During the past several years, we have had patients inform us that they did not go to the media because they were satisfied with our response to a medical error. We all would like to avoid our medical mishaps landing on the front page of the news – and, more importantly, we want to avoid the mishaps from occurring at all. Even when an event becomes the center of media attention, open and honest communication does not have to cease. During this past year, we have seen another major institution's CEO and physicians eloquently address and accept responsibility for a medical error that occurred at their facility by being more brutally open and honest about the situation than many of us would have anticipated. In the aftermath of a tragic medical error, this institution bared all and addressed the media head on. They could have taken a "no comment" approach to media inquiries, especially in light of potential litigation. However, the CEO and physicians not only acknowledged that an error had occurred, they described the details of the error and accepted responsibility for what had happened as a result of "human errors and an inefficient backup system." They even went a step further and publicly shared details of the occurrence and the actions they were taking as a result of their "sentinel review." Additionally, this institution has continued to share its ongoing reviews and results of external surveys with the public on its web site, long after the error has appeared in the news. I don't know of many institutions that have been this open, not only with the patient's family, but with the public.

Several years ago, the Cook County Bureau of Health Services had a case at one of its institutions that many felt marked the beginning of our departure from "the less said, the better" approach in dealing with medical errors. That case was similar to the FCH scenario in that after the family was informed of the unanticipated outcome, it was discovered that a medical error had occurred. Our clinicians were not speculating about the cause of the error, they were 99% sure that the error caused the patient's injury. The physicians were sure that once the patient's family got over the initial shock of what had happened, they would ask questions as to the cause of the injury and they needed to know how to respond to the family. In this case, it was decided that the chairman of the department, who had a wonderful rapport with patients, would speak to the family and tell them the truth as we knew it. This decision was not made lightly, since many staff were concerned that litigation would follow. But we decided that we would not be frozen by a fear of litigation, or whether our conversations with the family would be used against us in a lawsuit. Our words were the truth. Our staff continued to be open in their communications with the patient's family during the duration of the patient's hospitalization. We felt that the family could still trust us and our capability to skillfully care for the patient, despite what had occurred.

We are still working on being comfortable with being open with our communications with patients, physicians, and hospital staff. As a governmental institution, we are trying to change a decades' old stereotype of operating under an aura of secrecy. Individually, we are also working on being secure with our communication skills; we are discussing distressing situations with patients, and their families, to a degree that we have never done before. That is why we have a team of professionals who are skilled and experienced in communicating adverse outcomes with patients, that includes the Risk Management Director, Medical Director, Attending Physician, Nursing Director and others involved in formulating our response to the patient. In these difficult situations, we usually choose an experienced senior attending physician (usually the division or department chairman) to initially meet with the family.

In subsequent meetings with the patient, it has not been uncommon for the medical director and COO or other senior staff members to be present.

As part of FCH's response to medical errors, the CEO should ensure that this case is immediately referred to the appropriate Quality Review Committee established by the hospital and medical staff where a root-cause analysis should be performed. There are many questions to be answered here, such as:

- What actually occurred at the time the patient was undergoing the cardiac catheterization?
- When did the equipment malfunction?
- How quickly was it recognized?
- Who was doing the procedure?
- How did staff know that the equipment was defective?
- Did they have prior problems or was the equipment subject to a manufacturer, FDA, or other product alert or recall?

All of these questions will need to be answered in order to get to the true cause of the problem.

In the future, the CEO should avoid the immediate knee-jerk reaction to fire the involved employees. If he wants to take immediate action, then stop using the defective machine involved, and take any other similar machines out of service until a thorough clinical or biomedical engineering inspection has been performed. The response to immediately fire individuals is typical of the "name and blame" response. Although an investigation may reveal that "individual, versus system" problems were the ultimate cause of this event, it is premature to fire the employees until the true cause is known. It is the rare instance that employee failure is the sole cause of error. Although under certain circumstances, it may be prudent to suspend an employee from duty pending the investigation, if you fire the employee, you may be eliminating your best source of information needed to solve the real problem. Instead, most employees directly involved in a tragic error are usually devastated by what occurred, and are in need of support. The hospital should have a mechanism for referring such employees to an employee assistance program.

In summary, it appears that FCH had a partial system in place for internal and external reporting of information related to medical errors. The patient's family was informed of the unanticipated outcome and the CEO was promptly informed of the event as well. The CEO also involved his Director of Media Relations to handle external reporting of this event. However, their reporting system is incomplete, since quality assurance committees and other external entities (state, professional liability carrier, etc.) to which the hospital may be required to make an immediate report to are not included in this information loop. If this hospital wants to maintain its stellar reputation, the methods that the CEO is using to respond to medical errors need a major overhaul fast.

12

Ineffectual governance: Pleasant Valley Regional Health System

Pleasant Valley Regional Health System was a highly regarded, successful multi-hospital system in the Southeast. Tim Wiseman had been the CEO of Pleasant Valley for over eighteen years and had overseen its growth from a free-standing, general hospital into its current integrated system. In addition to its original hospital, Pleasant Valley now boasted a pediatric hospital, several strategically located primary care centers, an outpatient surgi-center, and an outpatient mental health facility. Pleasant Valley also enjoyed the services of a highly skilled, hospital-based group practice that included primary care physicians as well as specialists and subspecialists.

Tim was proud of his accomplishments over the last decade, and his governing board as well as the community at large regarded him with respect and admiration. Tim had a comfortable relationship with his board. Its deference to Tim was reflected in his astonishing track record in gaining the board's approval of every recommendation that he brought to them. Tim was grateful for the support that the board afforded him. He knew he was the envy of colleagues who often spoke of their boards' inability to differentiate between management and governance. Tim's board was willing to let him take the lead and it was quick to put its stamp of approval on his policy recommendations as well as his proposals for the growth and expansion of the organization.

Lately, however, Tim had been troubled by his board's unquestioning support. It seemed as though the burden of responsibility for Pleasant Valley rested squarely on Tim's shoulders and the weight of it was gnawing at him. As healthcare delivery became more and more complex, Tim came to realize how helpful it would be to have know-ledgeable, visionary board members to provide him with guidance and to share respon-sibility for the healthcare system's future.

The Pleasant Valley Board numbered thirty and, like many contemporary governing boards, was self-perpetuating. The average age of its members was sixty-five years, a figure that would have been lower had it not been for Ben Woodslea, well into his eighties, who had served on the board for over twenty years. Ben was a likeable gentleman who enjoyed the "perks and the prestige" of being a member of the Pleasant Valley Board. Indeed, the same could be said for several other board members, many of whom had

Management Mistakes in Healthcare, ed. Paul Hofmann and Frankie Perry. Published by Cambridge University Press. © Cambridge University Press 2005.

become close personal friends over the years and often socialized outside of the hospital setting.

Truth to tell, the board as a whole had contributed little to the success of the organization. In fact, the immediate past chairman had been heard to say, "The job of this board is to make sure we have a good CEO and then to stay out of his way." Tim had smiled when he first heard this, but now it annoyed him that the board was so ill-prepared to hold informed discussions on issues of significant import to Pleasant Valley. Tim had tried to provide the board with sufficient background information to generate meaningful deliberations, but to no avail. Comprehensive informational packets were delivered to the membership two weeks prior to each board meeting, and it was frustrating to watch a few of the members open those sealed packets upon their arrival at the meeting.

Tim knew he needed to recommend to the board leadership that they seriously evaluate the board's role and responsibilities in governing the organization. Several board retreats over the years had attempted to address this issue, and Tim had persuaded the board to engage the services of a respected consultant to lead these discussions. The board had even appointed a committee to study the evaluation process and make recommendations to strengthen it. A strong evaluation tool resulted from this effort, but the evaluation process itself was so perfunctory that it rendered the tool useless. Contributing to the problem was the size of the board, which tended to make it somewhat unwieldy.

Over the years, the organization had been successful and Tim had been very busy seeing to it that it was. He knew these governance issues were important if the organization was to continue to thrive and he knew he must deal with these issues sooner or later. For the time being, he had let them slide while he tended to what he considered more pressing needs of the organization. The Pleasant Valley Board was content to play out its current role in support of management. Individual board members were quite content as well, as long as their influence brought favor to friends and family in need of healthcare. Of necessity, Tim had designated a senior-level administrator to follow up on the multiple requests from board members that special attention be given to those of their acquaintance.

Tim's most immediate problem related to the board, however, was reining in what he considered to be some unreasonable expenses submitted by board members who attended a recent trustee symposium in Palm Springs. When Tim had approached Maryanne Metric, the board chair, with these expense reports, Maryanne had dismissed Tim's concerns with a shrug. From past experience, Tim knew that board members, even chairman-officers, were reluctant to be critical of one another. When it came to matters such as these, the board was a predictably cohesive group who viewed such things as expense reports as falling within its exclusive domain. Acutely aware of this, Tim had requested that the board develop and enforce a policy allowing only prudent and reasonable expenses, and that policy was about to be put to the test. Tim was annoyed that he had to spend valuable time on such matters when significant strategic decisions required attention.

Pleasant Valley had always enjoyed the lion's share of the market in its service area. But its position of dominance was being threatened by an influx of managed care plans into the geographic area. A significant number of provider contracts had been negotiated with competitors, and Pleasant Valley's market share appeared to be dwindling. To Tim's surprise, the Pleasant Valley Board had taken a firm position that it would not negotiate with "insurance companies" and would not discount services regardless of what the competition did.

As an alternative strategy, Tim met with the Executive Committee of the Board and suggested that Pleasant Valley explore the possibility of purchasing its own health plan. Tim argued that Pleasant Valley, with its strong primary care base and its large group practice, was well positioned to consider this. He proposed to engage the services of a managed care consultant to study the issue. Before bringing this recommendation to the board as a whole, he sought the support of the Executive Committee. The Executive Committee was appalled at this suggestion. Pleasant Valley was in the healthcare business, not in the "insurance business." The chairman-elect regaled the committee with his family's unfortunate experiences with HMOs up north. It was suggested that even exploring such a possibility could tarnish the reputation of Pleasant Valley.

It became abundantly clear to Tim that any reasonable discussion of the options available to Pleasant Valley at this juncture must follow extensive education to bring the board up to speed in the financing and delivery of healthcare in the managed care environment. Otherwise, their opinions would be those generated as a result of watching television news-magazine programs. Tim knew he must act quickly before managed care became a dead issue at Pleasant Valley. Informal discussions among board members would be less than informed. The opinions of physicians would be sought. It was more than likely that they would equate managed care with socialized medicine. In the past, board decisions had often fallen prey to the "group think syndrome." Tim had not encouraged the board to behave otherwise because this had always worked to his advantage. Now he wasn't so sure that this had been a smart practice on his part.

Commentary

Joyce A. Godwin

Tim Wiseman, in his role as CEO of Pleasant Valley Regional Health System (Pleasant Valley), is experiencing what many executives face all too often in their personal and professional lives. Things are going well. Sure, there could be some improvements, but the realities of time and place require attention to the urgent demands of the situation. Why mess with something that is good – even if it could become great? After all, might the situation not get worse? Why expend all the time and energy to take to the next level something that is okay as is?

In work, marriage, child rearing, social relationships, community activities, and recreational pursuits, this situation occurs more often than we choose to admit. We do the *urgent* at the expense of the *important*. We look for the easy answer, the quick fix, so we can get on to the next thing needing our urgent attention. We celebrate crossing off our lists each one of these "things" we fixed even though many of them wind up back on our lists for yet another quick fix. At the same time, success can breed complacency. From the viewpoint of those external to the organization or to the situation, they see what appears to be a problem-free career, a successful organization, an enviable relationship with the board, a great marriage, perfect families, sports trophies, acclaim in the community. They do not see, nor do we, how the "important" has taken back seat to the "urgent." They do not see that the "good" is all too often the enemy of what could be "great." While it is recognized that it is good to be challenged by people who can sharpen our thinking, who can provide stimulating discussions on alternate strategies, who can provoke us to think "outside of the box," or who can challenge us to challenge our boards, success often pushes these precepts aside. Although there are people with whom we can test new ideas and approaches, people who are committed to working with us to ratchet up our personal and organizational excellence to achieve "greatness," and success frequently means that these people are not sought out.

Such was the career of Tim Wiseman: over eighteen years at Pleasant Valley, over eighteen "successful" years with significant growth of the system and a board that had not set up roadblocks, but gave Tim a clear road ahead. His was a board that didn't interfere in management; and yet, it was a board that had become a complacent, rubber-stamp board, a board that majored in the minors, the "inconsequentials," a board that was too large, stale, and inbred. It was a board that seemed to be "in it" for the wrong reasons – the perks and prestige – for what being on a hospital board could do for them and their friends. It was an "old school" board from the time when it was a matter of prestige and privilege to be on the board of the local hospital, when that institution coveted listing the names of all the community leaders on its letterhead, when being on the hospital board meant getting special attention for family and friends, attending an occasional meeting to enjoy a good lunch or dinner with colleagues and hear a report about all the good things happening at the hospital. Meetings were to tell board members about the new innovations at the hospital so they could pass on the information at their service clubs, country clubs, and church get-togethers.

Changing times

Tim saw that times were changing, but had been unsuccessful in getting key board leaders or board members to move from dealing with the minors to dealing with the majors – to recognize the need for taking a good look at Pleasant Valley's *strategic direction and governance.* Ignored or unacknowledged was the need for Pleasant Valley to examine how it could maintain or even enhance the successes of the past, given the managed care environment in which it would be competing . . . and thriving or failing.

There is much to be learned from the critical things Tim did and did not do in his eighteen years at Pleasant Valley:

- How could Tim have avoided or prevented the situation in which he now finds himself?
- What can Tim do to get out of that situation?
- What risks do the Pleasant Valley board members themselves face, and what steps can Tim take to get the attention of his board members?
- How can Tim help his board provide through responsible governance the leadership needed to ensure that Pleasant Valley remains a strong and viable player in the changing healthcare market?

Management failures

Looking through the "retrospectoscope," we can see things Tim could have done differently. How did Tim get to where he is today? Certainly, Tim's failure to challenge his board to challenge him contributed to the board's complacency that now seems entrenched. Had Tim been advising his board effectively of the changing face of healthcare and financing, the chances are that he would not now be faced with a board that refuses to recognize the need to partner with insurance companies or to become otherwise involved in shaping a future that includes managed care. Without the combined commitment of management and board to challenging and open discussion, there is little likelihood that critical issues will be subject to a comprehensive hearing, debate, and resolution. Good management cannot succeed without good governance, something Pleasant Valley sorely needs. Tim's relationship with his board has been comfortable . . . too comfortable, and Tim bears some responsibility for promoting the board's "old school" attitude.

Tim made a couple of key mistakes. First, by designating a senior-level administrator to handle the board's requests for special favors for family and friends, Tim was working around two significant problems rather than confronting them. Board members are not there to seek and expect favors – and, more importantly, if those favors seem needed, isn't something wrong with the system? Why should a friend or acquaintance of a Pleasant Valley board member need special favors when they use the facilities and services of the health system? Is this because Pleasant Valley is not the highly regarded health system it is perceived to be? Should these requests for special favors not be a signal to both Tim and the board that all is not well, that every patient and guest at Pleasant Valley is not a "special person?" Tim did not address this situation directly. He taught board members that getting special favors for friends and family was not only one of their perks, it was so important that Tim assigned a senior member of management to facilitate this expectation. Tim was rewarding board members for inappropriate behavior and such behavior had become *institutionalized.*

Second, and more importantly, Tim allowed his board to take a back seat, rubber-stamping his decisions. Tim's eighteen years of nurturing a board that would "get out of his way" has resulted in the situation now facing him and Pleasant Valley: a *lack of leadership* at a time when leadership is most needed. Tim cannot simply point fingers at the board and its leadership. A board will be only as good as management will help it become. Tim and the board may have been rationalizing through its years of unchallenged success . . . and, like most of us, their ability to rationalize had no upper limit. Tim now realizes that he needs the guidance and support of a fully engaged board to help Pleasant Valley overcome the challenges it faces; instead, Tim has a board that provides no "value added." The board is made up of "takers," not "givers." It functions as a social club both in and out of board meetings. "Let Tim do it" has become not a celebration of Tim's success but the board's excuse for abdicating its responsibilities.

To his credit, Tim has tried a number of things to get the board engaged, such as providing background information to generate meaningful deliberations, holding retreats, engaging a respected consultant to evaluate the board's role and responsibilities in governing Pleasant Valley, developing a strong board evaluation tool, having trustees attend symposia, and meeting with the Executive Committee, to develop support for bringing a recommendation to the full board. These are many good, appropriate actions. But all of these efforts have failed to produce meaningful action on the part of the board.

Why have these efforts failed? Let us assume there is a pen on the table. If someone says to you, "Try to move it," how do you go about "trying" to move the pen? You can't will the pen to move. You either reach out and move it or you don't. Or when more innovative "out of the box" solutions are required, you move the pen by moving the table. But that's moving the pen – not "trying." You cannot simply try. If you are committed to "trying," you will be sitting there for a long time. If you are committed to "doing," that pen can move quickly. Although Tim had tried many things, he had achieved no results. The board did not "move."

But has Tim really challenged the board? Has he developed a clear, no-holds barred presentation to the board, painting a picture of the likely scenario for Pleasant Valley if the board does not come to grips with the changes in healthcare? Has he hit hard on the board members' fiduciary responsibilities and the potential liabilities the individual board members may face if the hospital fails to thrive? Has Tim clearly described how Pleasant Valley's current board differs in any number of ways from the boards needed to guide today's healthcare systems? Has he spoken of the board members' unquestioning support over the years, but pointed out that now, if Pleasant Valley is not to further lose market share, he needs not only their support but also a knowledgeable, visionary board that can be an "iron sharpens iron" body for him and Pleasant Valley? Has he told the board that he wants to make it his priority to work with them to facilitate the board's transition into the body Pleasant Valley needs not only now, but also for its future? Through a strong challenge, has Tim motivated the board or even frightened them into action?

Tim also seems to have missed the opportunity to develop leadership in Pleasant Valley's medical staff. Pleasant Valley enjoys the services of a highly skilled, hospital-based group practice that included primary care physicians, as well as specialists and subspecialists. Nonetheless, Tim suspected that if the board solicited their opinions, these physicians would be unable to speak knowledgeably about the challenges of managed care and how Pleasant Valley could – and must – compete with the new players in its market. Before Tim brought these issues to the board, he should have worked with the Pleasant Valley medical staff to help them to understand managed care and Pleasant Valley's competitive current and future environments. The current situation raises a number of major questions.

- Has Tim considered seeking out a well-respected physician or small group of physicians to champion an *objective look* at managed care – what managed care would mean for the Pleasant Valley medical staff and the future of the health system?
- Has Tim seriously discussed with medical staff leaders the need to *contract with insurers or even purchase a health plan?*
- Has he brought in *previously doubting or antagonistic-to-managed-care physicians* who have been "transformed" from systems with characteristics similar to Pleasant Valley?
- Has he supported the formation of a *task force of physician leaders,* combined with board members who do not rely solely on television news-magazine programs for their healthcare intelligence, to determine how Pleasant Valley could best address managed care?
- Has he developed *scenarios* of what likely would happen if the board (a) maintained its current stance, (b) pursued managed care, or (c) prepared another strategy to assure the continued market share of Pleasant Valley?

- Has he visited colleagues in *similar markets* who had successfully wrestled with managed care issues?

It seems clear now that Pleasant Valley management failed to educate both its board and its medical staff on an ongoing basis. As a result, Pleasant Valley is now in a *reactive mode* and the position of dominance it has enjoyed will quickly become history if fast and responsible action is not taken.

If Tim has really challenged the board, and has engaged the medical staff in his vision, does he have any options if the board still does not step up to its responsibilities? The answer is "yes." Sometimes the unusual must be done to experience the incredible.

Might Tim take the bold step of sending a letter to the board in which he clearly articulates the problem(s) and indicates that unless the board commits to quickly and seriously addressing these issues and developing an action plan to resolve them that Tim believes the board should begin the process of identifying a new CEO – one who will be comfortable in maintaining the status quo? Career-limiting action, one might say. Yes, but why should a competent CEO stay in a situation in which the board is not stepping up to its responsibilities? Tim, an experienced healthcare executive, is seeing what he has built over the last eighteen years being eroded by a board unwilling to even explore the changing healthcare environment. He's also seeing that he has failed to develop a strong board – one that can help him and Pleasant Valley grow and prosper. He has grown accustomed to the lack of challenge and oversight, and even enjoyed these things for a number of years. In many ways, today's board is a product of the relationship that Tim has permitted to exist. It appears as if the Pleasant Valley board is on the slippery slope from good to mediocre to non-performing. And Tim has been greasing the skids of that slippery slope.

Tim has to make a decision. In his relationship with the board, does Tim want to continue being a conformer, or does he want to be a transformer?

Governance failures

Like Tim, a well-informed board member should be asking why she should stay on a board that is not fulfilling its fiduciary responsibilities. Why invest time preparing for and attending meetings in which the expectation and desired actions are just more "rubber-stamping?" Might there not be another organization that could better use and appreciate their time and talents? It seems that the Pleasant Valley board members have not been oriented appropriately about their responsibilities as board members. Perhaps they are not knowledgeable about their Duty of Care, their Duty of Inquiry, their Duty of Loyalty, and their Duty of Prudent Investment, how to fulfill these duties, or the consequences of failing to fulfill these duties. Perhaps they have not been briefed on the implications of Sarbanes–Oxley or how to deal with real and perceived conflicts of interest. The self-perpetuating nature of the board indicates that Pleasant Valley is a non-profit healthcare system. Do the board members understand issues of private inurement and private benefit, and the risk of personal liability for Intermediate Sanctions? Perhaps the Pleasant Valley board has not taken seriously the requirements of corporate compliance programs and the meaning and importance of HIPAA and other key healthcare laws and regulatory compliance issues. Perhaps the Pleasant Valley board remains unaware of the allegations of attorneys general throughout the country that the "waste of charitable assets" by management and by boards require redress. Perhaps the board is oblivious to the fact that the rules of governance have changed – and are still evolving. Healthcare organizations, in particular, are operating in an environment of heightened responsibility, scrutiny, and regulation. What is going on with the Pleasant Valley board? Ignorance? Benign neglect? Laziness? An experienced healthcare executive like Tim should be asking himself these same questions.

While it is not uncommon for a board to have a crisis of confidence in the CEO or leadership team, it is probably more unusual for a CEO or leadership team to have a crisis of confidence in the board. If Tim elects to write the "shake 'em up" letter to the board, what should the letter say? It should be simple and straight forward, enumerating his concerns and the board's lack of response. Tim can say that he has failed in bringing about a strong governance process for Pleasant Valley, that he deeply regrets and assumes responsibility for this failure. The letter should not go into the detailed problems or potential solutions; let the magnitude of Tim's message sink in. A concerned board would want to call a special meeting to explore in more depth his concerns and the board's plan of action. Should the board not take seriously Tim's concerns and his statement that he had not succeeded in bringing about a governance system using best practices, that would be a powerful signal to Tim that it was time to move on.

If the board wishes to step up to its responsibilities, reflecting on the excellence of their CEO over the last eighteen years and believing that he might have some valid concerns about the future of Pleasant Valley, what might be an appropriate course of action? First, the board must *assume ownership* of the problem and the opportunity. It would be highly preferable to work first on the governance transformation, out of which could emerge a board with the members and the mandate to position Pleasant Valley to compete and thrive in the new healthcare environment.

Governance transformation and redesign

The board should first determine that it is prepared to quickly, but comprehensively, address its own lack of governance, in both process and substance. This would include identifying best practices in corporate and healthcare governance and studying, understanding, adopting, and implementing those appropriate for Pleasant Valley. That this is a time-intensive undertaking, requiring considerable work from board leadership and management and staff, must be clearly understood and accepted.

If Pleasant Valley does not have the luxury of time to structure a comprehensive plan for its future governance, due to Tim's concerns about the encroachment of managed care, the organization must work on understanding and implementing best practices in governance while appreciating and addressing its managed care environment. Proceeding on these parallel tracks will take an even bigger commitment on the part of the board and management.

Working with Tim, the board leadership can schedule a series of special sessions in which to explore background information on best practices in governance and to develop an understanding of the current and anticipated impact of managed care in their service area. Perhaps a "board champion" could emerge for each of the two areas. The champions would work closely with Tim, on behalf of the board, to see that plans were expedited for bringing information and recommendations to the board. When discussing managed care, selected members of the medical staff with a balanced view and not perpetuators of "war stories" should be invited as guests to the board meeting.

Managed care

Working with his colleagues across the country, Tim can identify and explore service areas with characteristics similar to those of Pleasant Valley. Ideally, there would be examples of systems that strategically planned for and addressed managed care as well as ones that had had tragic business consequences because of their shortsightedness. Board chairs or other appropriate representatives of such organizations could be asked to address the Pleasant Valley board, and possibly the medical staff or its leadership, about their experiences. If it could not be arranged for the chairs of these boards to visit Pleasant Valley, then perhaps a delegation from the Pleasant Valley board and a few physicians might visit their counterparts elsewhere. Should these visits take place, it is important that Tim provide comprehensive information to the other CEO and board leadership about Pleasant Valley's current position, as it relates to its governance practices and to managed care, so that the visiting or visited colleagues can make their observations as relevant as possible.

There could be local resources – other for-profit or not-for-profit entities – that have gone through governance restructuring and could share their journeys with the Pleasant Valley board. Much can be learned from the experiences, both positive and negative, of others, whether in healthcare or other industries.

To be effective in this endeavor, Tim must understand how his board members best *learn*. For some board members and medical staff leaders, presenting journal articles or case studies in written or audio format might be helpful. Others may prefer to watch videos and some may be more comfortable exploring recommended web sites or doing their own Internet research. Others need to hear from colleagues one on one. Still others need to see in person what is going on in another market. Providing an audiotape to someone who never listens to tapes is a waste of time; likewise, providing the best book available on a given subject to board members who are not readers is a waste of time and money. Tim needs to understand how his board members and medical staff leaders learn, so that he can provide the tools that work for them.

Tim also needs to be wary of a too-quick response to "Let's have a consultant come in here and help us." Pleasant Valley's board members must first commit to personally addressing governance practices and managed care in their service area. Bringing in a consultant before the board takes full ownership of the problem or the opportunity is premature. Board members first need to understand the magnitude of what's before them. A "quick fix" will be just that. The tendency to delegate the problem and solution to a consultant must be avoided. Tim previously brought in consultants and it proved to be useless when the board failed to recognize the problem at hand. Work also needs to progress on projecting Pleasant Valley's future financials, especially if the Executive Committee maintains its position of not being in the "insurance business." Ideally, the board should request that financial forecasts be prepared while other governance and managed care work is in progress.

"Intentionality" is the key word in proceeding on both the governance and managed care tracks. There must be full "buy in" to the concerns, opportunities, and work plan. There must be commitment to move ahead as a body. As previously indicated, it would be best first to address the governance concerns; but there may not be the luxury of time to do that well and in a manner in which it will be positively received and implemented, given the immediate need to address the managed care "crisis."

Current board members must understand from the beginning that addressing Tim's concerns will involve a significant time commitment, in and out of board meetings, as individuals, and as a body. This time commitment applies whether board members decide to seriously address Tim's concerns or whether they find themselves in the business of searching for a new CEO. This is a good and convenient time to encourage board members who do not have the time, interest, or expertise to devote to this "crisis," to resign from the board. Make it very acceptable for people to resign; recognize and celebrate their tenure on the board. This can be a first and immediate step in getting the board to a more manageable size, even before best governance practices are studied, determined, and imple-mented. A board of a more manageable size will facilitate meaningful deliberations about managed care. Of course, care needs to be taken that the most qualified current board members are not the ones who wish to resign. Too often the people already understanding their responsibilities and working to fulfill them are the ones who think they are not doing enough.

Governance structure and reformation

On the governance track, the "board champion" and a couple of board colleagues might work with Tim on an action plan for the board. Identifying systems that have implemented governance best practices is helpful. Communicating with other systems about their "whys" and "hows" can be beneficial. And, as seen above, visits can be very useful. Likewise, Tim can identify boards that have been closer in governance practices to Pleasant Valley's "old-school" ways but have been through some type of a "board crisis" – bankruptcy, extensive legal action in which it was clear that the board had not fulfilled its fiduciary responsibilities or had had conflicts of interest, etc. Unfortunately, some boards and their members need to be frightened into action.

It is important that when a board becomes committed to reforming itself and implementing best practices, it does so for the right reasons. In this case, the board's motivation must not be just to apply a few band-aids to keep Tim around and get over the current crisis. The board, individually and as a body, must become committed to a *philosophy and action plan for excellence* in *governance* as a means of promoting excellence throughout Pleasant Valley Regional Health System.

An early demonstration of the board's commitment to "reform itself" would be for it to take responsibility for enforcing its own *expense policy*. If the board needs a little prodding on this, perhaps a board member who was at the Palm Springs symposium could paint a picture for his or her colleagues of how the expenses would look on the front page, above the centerfold, of the local newspaper. With the corporate governance and accounting scandals of the early 2000s, there exists a plethora of excellent material on implementing best governance practices. There also exist plenty of headlines and television news-magazines programs to remind Pleasant Valley of what happens when board members are not "minding" the store. Might some of these just be the Pleasant Valley Regional Health System on a larger scale?

We don't know whether Pleasant Valley has ever considered a governance format in which business groups of the system – such as the tertiary care hospital, pediatric hospital, physician practices, outpatient service (primary care centers, surgi-center), and mental health facility, or some logical clustering of these busi-ness units – would have their own boards of trustees reporting to a system board of directors. The pros and cons of such a structure could be appropriately explored during this period of intense focus on Pleasant Valley's current and future governance. Should there be good business reasons for such a governance structure, the "abolishment" of the current thirty-person board might be more palatable to several of its current members. Should the above not be pursued, for whatever reason, intense work needs to commence on reforming the "one board for all business units" structure.

The board could request Tim to resurrect the work previously done on board roles and responsibilities, to determine whether that work might be useful as a starting point for the board's commitment to becoming serious about them. Just reviewing this document should make clear that the board's responsibility is considerably more than, "Make sure we have a good CEO and then stay out of his way." Likewise, the evaluation tool could be resurrected for later potential use. Before it's used again, however, there would be many prerequisites, including a discussion on:

- Why evaluate?
- Who will assume leadership and follow through of the process?
- What will we do with the results?

A *draft work plan* for the board's governance redesign needs to be prepared for the board's deliberation, modification, or acceptance. Perhaps that senior-level administrator now in charge of "favors for board members" might be redeployed to do some more appropriate staff work for the board. Where is Tim going to get the time to provide the necessary personal leadership and diligence to assist with the board's commitment to bring about a new governance system? It is likely that he will need to delegate some of the less important "urgent" matters that are easier to address so he can focus on the more difficult and important issues.

Following the defining of the board's role and responsibilities, care should be taken to design the *ideal board* – not "who" but how many people, with what characteristics and abilities, are needed to govern Pleasant Valley? The board will have to come to grips with the fact that their current thirty-member set-up is too large. There can be creative ways, however, to get the governing body down to a more appropriate size of nine–thirteen members, without sacrificing some type of relationship with Pleasant Valley for those individuals who want to maintain their affiliation. The new board, regardless of the final size determined to be most efficient and effective for governing Pleasant Valley, should comprise some new members, as well as some of the more qualified individuals from the current board. It is best for all thirty members of the current board to submit letters of resignation. Some current board members would probably want to make clear that they do not wish to be considered for the new board; a few who have served for many years and with distinction, assuming Pleasant Valley had some of these, could become emeritus board members, if the by-laws provide such an honor. If emeritus board members are named, care must be taken to clarify that these people will not be attending board meetings or participating in the governance process, but that they will receive special communications from the CEO and be invited to some of the board's social functions. Other current board members might serve on some special task forces in the future or serve on a President's Council in which they would be invited to have lunch at one of the Pleasant Valley facilities, get an update on current and upcoming happenings at the health system, receive reports from the CEO, and provide feedback to the President about the community's perceptions of Pleasant Valley. These sessions could be scheduled on a semi-annual or more frequent basis, as need for this type of communication warrants.

By-laws must be reviewed and rewritten to reflect all the changes that will be made to the governance of Pleasant Valley. Particular attention needs to be given to whether there will be term limits and age limits, and what committees the board will have.

Term and age limits

To expedite the work for Tim and the Pleasant Valley board, a few recommendations and commentary follow. As so much of the current and continuing "governance reformation process" will fall under the Governance Committee, expanded recommendations and commentary appear for this group.

Term limits

A term of three years, with the possibility of being *nominated* to serve up to three successive terms is recommended. (Note: *nominated*, not re-elected). In no way should a current board member assume that renomination or re-election is automatic. Rather, the board's needs at the conclusion of a member's three-year term must be considered, along with the board member's interest in continuing, their past and potential future contributions, and their ability to devote the requisite time to their board responsibilities. The Governance Committee (see below) would have responsibility for this process of consideration for renomination. A board member who has served three successive terms, followed by one or more years off, could be considered for renomination should he or she so desire and should the Pleasant Valley board need someone with that individual's skills and potential contributions. The one-year "sabbatical" provides a great opportunity for evaluation of the mutual interest in serving again. Should the individual be renominated and elected to serve, the returning board member comes with fresh ideas and new perspectives. This is a "win–win" situation. It is remarkable how seriously people take board service when there is a serious interview, nomination, election and evaluation process.

Age limits

With a good solid evaluation process and a commitment to diversity, including age, age limits should not be necessary. People of different generations think in different ways. Board deliberations are richer if diverse perspectives are part of the deliberations. Having a board totally comprised of people whose ages all fall within one decade is not diversity.

Recommended committees

Have as few as possible to get the job done. Some states will require that boards have certain committees, so care must be taken to understand state requirements. With a small board, there is no need for the use of an executive committee, although there may be a good reason to provide for one, such as for approving a bank resolution or something similar for which action is needed very quickly and for which the full board has already delegated responsibility. Routine use of an executive committee tends to disenfranchise members of the board who are not on the executive committee. Two classes of board members emerge, and a small board cannot afford to have any second-class citizens. With today's electronic means of communicating, there is little excuse for not being able to get in touch with the full board. Conference calls, e-mails, and faxes serve as excellent communication tools for when it's not feasible or warranted to bring together the board in person. It is important to be sure that the bylaws provide for communicating electronically.

Committees to establish

Many boards fail to operate effectively because they do not have appropriate committees with clearly described responsibilities. The brief descriptions that follow provide a general overview of the type of committees that should be established, and their functions.

Compliance and audit committee

This committee would have oversight of all of Pleasant Valley's compliance programs, as well as internal and external audits. In looking for candidates for the board, special care should be taken to think in terms of members and leaders for this committee, both currently and for the future. While these stipulations would not currently exist for Pleasant Valley, looking at the Sarbanes–Oxley Act, New York Stock Exchange (NYSE) and Securities and Exchange Commission (SEC) requirements for audit committee members is probably predictive of what will eventually be required by some financial or regulatory body to which Pleasant Valley is or will be subject. Preparing for that eventuality now is prudent. It will also provide more qualified compliance and audit committee members. Experience in regulatory environments, compliance programs, and risk management is another great background for members of this committee.

Finance committee

This committee would have responsibility for the on-going financial performance of Pleasant Valley, as well as reviewing and recommending the annual operating and capital budgets to the full board. Financing or refinancing of the Pleasant Valley system would come under this committee's purview. The committee would also assume responsibility for assessing the financial aspects of Pleasant Valley's strategic plan and exploring scenarios for being "in or out" of managed care. Pleasant Valley's investment portfolio could come under the purview of this committee, or the finance committee could appoint a subcommittee to oversee investments.

Governance committee

Oversight of Pleasant Valley's governance process rests here. This includes by-laws, job descriptions for board and committee members and officers, interviews of potential board candidates, nominations, evaluations, committee charters, board continuing education, governance manual, and best practices. The committee should establish universal competencies required of all board members and the collective competencies that should be available when the individual board members are seen as a body.

To assure the appropriate format and content for all minutes in the Pleasant Valley system, this committee should establish sample minutes and see that a seminar is held for everyone who has responsibility for preparing minutes. Too often, minutes are not properly prepared or reviewed prior to approval. When those approving minutes realize that when they approve minutes they are approving their deposition, care begins to be taken. Those not present at a meeting should abstain from approving the minutes of that meeting. Two signature lines with dates should be at the end of all minutes. The first is for the recording secretary or individual who submitted the minutes for approval. The second signature line is for the corporate secretary or chairman of the board or committee and is not affixed until the requisite body has taken action, including any amendments, on the minutes. It is too late when in court on a legal matter in which members of the Pleasant Valley board have been named to say: "Oh, I wasn't at that meeting when they decided that" when your name appears on the list of members present.

Quality committee

The board should want to establish quality goals that this committee would monitor and measure. Depending on how Pleasant Valley's medical staff is organized and what the by-laws indicate for privileging, credentialing, etc., this committee may take on some of these responsibilities. Just as the Governance committee will lead the board on a journey to excellence in governance, this committee will lead the board on a quality journey, such that all patients and guests at Pleasant Valley will receive the same excellent service previously assured for board members and their families and friends.

Guiding principles for the future

As considerable work is going to be required for Tim and the board on both the journey to excellence in governance and the study of managed care, the following alphabet highlights the most critical considerations on this specific trip and their future journeys together:

A *Absolute integrity* **between what you are thinking and what you are saying**

This is a must for not only the implementation of a governance system characterized by best practices and the study of managed care, but for all future board deliberations. Without absolute integrity between what is being said and what is being thought, endless misunderstandings, redo of work, and unnecessary expenditures of time to solve problems that should not have occurred will result.

B *Best practices*

Learn them and use them, not only for governance, but for how to tackle an issue such as the study of the pros and cons of managed care for Pleasant Valley.

C *Culture of excellence*

In governance and throughout Pleasant Valley, define what this means, establish goals and measurement tools to monitor progress. Have the board set the example for the health system.

D *Design* **for excellence**

When refining Pleasant Valley's by-laws, establishing board and committee job descriptions, committee charters, etc., keep excellence in mind. A fantastic opportunity exists when starting from scratch. The goal of excellence can be designed into the new documents and processes. Abolish mediocrity.

E *Evaluation, evaluation, evaluation*

In real estate, it's location, location, location. On Pleasant Valley's journey to excellence, it's evaluation, evaluation, evaluation. At the end of each committee and board meeting, at the end of each year, self-evaluations and board evaluations must be completed. What gets measured, gets improved.

F *Feelings*

Don't let feelings gets in the way of facts, especially on issues concerning people.

G *Governance principles*

Those who are invested in the stock market and receive proxies will note that increasingly corporations are listing their governance principles. This is in response to the recent corporate scandals, regulations, and literature on best practices. Reading proxies can further board members' governance education.

H *Honor the history* of the organization

Understand Pleasant Valley's history and the people responsible for its founding and development; honor them, but don't languish in the past. Be a leader in Pleasant Valley's "future history."

I *Interview* potential board candidates

Extensively interview people for a board of a voluntary organization, a not-for-profit organization, any organization? Yes, if you are serious about governance and want prospective board members to understand this. Requesting a résumé and presenting potential board candidates with a job description prior to an interview is essential. Discussing Pleasant Valley's expectations of board members in an interview with two members of the Governance committee and Tim will get the potential board member off to a great start. When potential candidates wish to be nominated after these steps, they know what they are getting into and will have arranged their schedules and other commitments so that they can serve Pleasant Valley well.

J *Just do it!*

Take responsibility for being part of the solution, rather than being part of the problem.

K *Know* the current and future membership needs in terms of skills, backgrounds, age diversity, constituencies, etc. of your board

You can then ensure that the existing and potential members serve the organization exceptionally well.

L *Look* for potential board members on an ongoing basis

In their various venues, board members should observe, make notes, and pass along to the Governance committee the names of potential candidates. The

Governance committee should be looking at board member and leadership needs three to six years out. Becoming aware of people who would bring excellence to the Pleasant Valley board is the job of all board members.

M   *Measure*

As noted previously, what gets measured, gets done. The board should, at each board meeting, monitor and measure progress on its compliance, financial condition, governance, quality, or whatever goals it establishes.

N   *Numbers*

"I don't do numbers" is a statement too often heard from members of boards, and it is not acceptable. All board members should be able to understand the balance sheet and the income and expense statement. As healthcare accounting does have some unique features, Pleasant Valley's monthly financial statements can be a good subject for a board education session.

O   *Organizations of complexity*

Healthcare organizations fit into this category. They have a large number of employees from those with minimal education to others with multiple degrees and specialties, including lots of people who think that their credentials indicate they do not need to follow internal and external regulations, and bureaucracies to handle the sheer magnitude of the operation. Look for at least one potential board member with experience in a complex organization. This can facilitate the board's understanding that it is not so simple to get things done in a complex organization. Tim will appreciate this support.

P   *Provocative discussions*

Frame the issues for board deliberations so that the experience and diversity of thinking on the board can be used to its full advantage.

Keep in mind that documents for governance decisions usually differ from documents for management decisions. Executive summaries are much appreciated.

Q   *Quality*

Make this the word that comes to mind whenever Pleasant Valley Regional Health System gets mentioned. Define what "quality" means for Pleasant Valley. Develop action plans, monitor progress, and celebrate success.

R   *Respect, trust, and candor in relationships*

Fulfilling this principle will determine whether the Pleasant Valley board will thrive or fail. With the reconstituted board having "new blood," as well as some previous board members, time needs to be set aside for everyone to get acquainted. People must know each other before they can respect each other. When they respect one another, they can trust one another. From this comes candor. From candor comes respect. The end result is excellence in Pleasant Valley board's deliberations and decision-making.

S   *Strategic plan*

This document is not one that goes on the bookshelf and gathers dust or gets lost, but is a living document continually used in Pleasant Valley's work. Each board meeting focuses on the strategy and considers modifications, if appropriate.

T   *Talking*

Asking questions, getting clarifications, participating in the board room and during meetings, not in covert "rump" sessions in the hallway or on the telephone after meetings.

U   *"Undiscussables"*

Identify "undiscussables" and get them on the table for discussion. On evaluations, ask for "undiscussables"; discuss and resolve them. Determine if there is a corporate culture in Pleasant Valley that says; "No one delivers bad news." If so, find out from where it emanates and make it clear that this is not acceptable, given the quality and excellence standards and values of Pleasant Valley. It can be extremely expensive if a "whistleblower" reports illegal practices to an external body because the "whistleblower" said that no one listened or wanted to hear bad news within the system.

V   *Values*

Determine these for your board – what are the absolutes? The board must have the moral values, maturity, and confidence to do what they know is right.

W   *WorldCom, Enron, Global Crossing, Tyco, etc.*

"There but for the grace of God go I?" Learn from these corporate failures. Recognize that these failures are not unique to large corporations.

X   *"Xchange"*

Exchange ideas with your counterparts at healthcare symposia. Meet with your colleagues at these conferences to determine which action plans you should develop or have on the agenda for your next board meeting. Good intentions often fall by the wayside when program participants return home.

Y *Yoke yourself to organizational improvement*

Make a dedicated commitment to improving personal skills, and an organizational culture that promotes continuous learning and development.

Z *Zero incidents of "I had no idea what they were talking about"*

Make a pledge to encourage clarification, ask questions, and to help board members understand the actions requiring their votes. Should legal action occur involving the Pleasant Valley board, it's then too late, too embarrassing, and too awkward to say, "But, I had no idea what they were talking about."

Tim and the board of Pleasant Valley have a great opportunity ahead of them *if* they individually and collectively want to follow these essential ABCs and confront what's before them. If not, then it's time for Tim to move on and take what he's learned from his eighteen years at Pleasant Valley to a new organization. Perhaps someone will be left at Pleasant Valley who can write the last chapter in its history – how a once great healthcare system died because of poor governance.

13

Failed hospital merger: Richland River Valley Healthcare System

The scenic Richland River meanders through historically prosperous Clay County. In the heart of this fertile valley lies the charming and picturesque city of Richland. The suburban area surrounding Richland, with its rolling hills and abundance of natural beauty, has attracted developers and now boasts elite resorts and retirement communities for the wealthy. The population of Clay County, including the city of Richland, is just under 500,000.

Clay County is proud of its healthcare services and touts them in its promotions to attract new industry to the area. The county has six hospitals, four within the city of Richland and two in the outlying suburban areas. Suburban Medical Center is a 150-bed general acute care hospital and Community Behavioral Health Center is a fifty-bed residential center with an innovative and highly regarded outpatient treatment center. Within the city of Richland, the well-respected major healthcare providers are Trinity Medical Center and Sutton Memorial Hospital. The other two general acute care hospitals within the city of Richland, both just under 200 beds, are not considered major players in the healthcare arena of Clay County. On the other hand, both Trinity and Sutton Memorial are the providers of choice for the vast majority of the population of Clay County.

While both of these organizations are well-respected providers of high-quality healthcare, they are very different in mission and structure. Trinity Medical Center is a faith-based organization that is part of a larger, regional religious system. Its mission is to care for those in need regardless of their ability to pay and as a result, Trinity provides the vast majority of indigent care within Clay County, and its programs have been developed in response to the needs of the younger population it tends to serve. Enormous resources have been committed to its high-risk Obstetrics program, Neonatal Intensive Care Unit, and its Pediatrics program with its attendant Pediatrics Intensive Care Unit. Trinity is also the designated Level I Trauma Center for the county and has committed considerable resources to its critical care programs that include a surgical and a medical intensive care unit and renal dialysis and burn units. In addition to its general medical–surgical units, it operates Oncology, Cardiology and Orthopedics programs, all supported with active outpatient clinics and rehabilitation programs. The professional personnel, especially the nurses, at Trinity are exceptionally loyal to the hospital and are highly skilled,

Management Mistakes in Healthcare, ed. Paul Hofmann and Frankie Perry. Published by Cambridge University Press. © Cambridge University Press 2005.

competent and compassionate. They are also unionized, but Trinity has implemented strong, effective management–employee programs and the unions are committed to the continued success of the Trinity organization.

The J. Blair Sutton Memorial Hospital is a privately owned, richly endowed healthcare organization; J. Blair Sutton was the founder of Sutton Manufacturing and Construction Inc., a company that brought great wealth to its founder and employment to many of the residents of Richland. The Sutton family is "old money" originally acquired from sawmills along the Richland River. J. Blair Sutton was quick to respond to modern technologies and when the time was right, he diversified his holdings and entered commercial construction and the manufacturing of doors, windows, and lumber products. That was in the 1940s, and the Sutton name and its products are now known nationwide. When it became the duty and obligation of the Sutton progeny to manage the family money, they moved from Richland to New York City, but the Sutton name still graces the streets of Richland, on schools, avenues, plazas, and prominent buildings throughout the community.

J. Blair Sutton Memorial Hospital is one such legacy. The 275-bed acute care hospital is renowned throughout the state for its cardiology services with its respected and successful open heart surgery program, its orthopedic surgery program specializing in hip replacements, and its cancer care program which has attracted nationally recognized oncologists and cancer surgeons. In addition to these "pillars of excellence," Sutton Memorial operates general medical–surgical, obstetrics, and pediatrics services, as well, but these programs command fewer resources at Sutton Memorial whose mission is to serve the healthcare needs of the "older families" of Clay County. The governing board of Sutton Memorial has no problem supporting this mission – after all, Trinity very capably and compassionately cares for the indigent in Clay County. It is Sutton Memorial's mission to provide healthcare for those who continue to commit their personal wealth to enrich the Richland community. This philosophy is in keeping with J. Blair Sutton's personal philosophy, deeply rooted in American capitalism and the right of the individual to reap the rewards and privileges of his hard work. His philosophy did not abide government intervention of any manner and in keeping with this, the Sutton Memorial board did all that it could for as long as it could to legally avoid caring for Medicare and Medicaid patients, operating on a cash basis until the recent past. This was very appealing to the members of the Sutton Memorial board, the majority of whom are corporate executives with companies of international stature, recruited to the board by the influential Sutton family.

In contrast, the Trinity governing board comprises representatives of the community, the religious order, and local bank, and corporate executives. These two governing boards, very different in philosophy, have little reason to interact with one another. They do not travel in the same social circles and the Sutton Memorial board members are most often back running their corporations in other states. The Sutton Memorial board meets quarterly, while the Trinity board, with its local members, meets monthly. The administrations of the two organizations seem content to maintain the status quo – after all, both organizations are operating well. Strong governing boards at each of these hospitals have made it clear to their respective CEOs that their jobs are to manage operations. In spite of their differences, the two organizations amicably co-exist in the city of Richland, each successful in its own right.

But all of that was about to change. In the 1990s, the national for-profit hospital corporations began to emerge as a force in healthcare. Indeed, Continental Healthcare, one of these, began purchasing private, not-for-profit hospitals in Clay County. One of the smaller hospitals in the city of Richland had already been purchased by Continental which has entered into negotiations with Suburban Medical Center. Both Trinity and Sutton Memorial were alarmed and fearful of losing their positions of prominence within Clay County. After much separate discussion, the governing boards at each hospital arrived at the same conclusion; they needed to partner with another organization to shore up their position within the community. As each organization sought an appropriate partner, it became clear all they had was each other.

The governing boards of the two organizations took the lead in exploring the merger of Trinity and Sutton Memorial. The administrations of the two organizations were only minimally involved and for the most part, remained focused on daily operations. Each governing board engaged the services of a different consultant to explore the feasibility of the merger. Following the consultants' report, both Trinity and Sutton Memorial decided it was in the best interests of their respective organizations for the two to merge into a single system. At this point the two governing boards first met for a face-to-face discussion, during which it was decided to jointly engage the services of a nationally known consulting firm with experience in successfully implementing the mergers of healthcare organizations. The consultant's report clearly laid out the enormous benefits, both present and future, which would accrue to both organizations once the merger was fully implemented. This report evolved into the only "strategic plan" used by the newly merged system and showed a savings of millions of dollars by merging business operations and sharing expensive medical technology. The report also promised the merger would increase bargaining power with health plans.

An initial step in the process was to determine the asset value of each organization. It was determined that Trinity assets were valued $25 million more than those of Sutton Memorial. In order for the two organizations to enter into the merger as equal partners, Trinity placed $25 million into a newly created foundation for the merged system, named the Richland River Valley Healthcare System (RRVHS) to use for healthcare programs in Clay County. Although agreeing with this resolution, the Sutton Memorial board was visibly annoyed with the results of the asset valuation. It was clear its members were unaccustomed to being second best at anything.

As the implementation of the merger moved forward, it was agreed the RRVHS governing board would number twenty-five: twelve members from Trinity, twelve members from Sutton Memorial and the new RRVHS CEO. The RRVHS board would be responsible for strategic planning and financial oversight of the system. Sutton Memorial would appoint the board chair for a two-year term; Trinity would then appoint the succeeding board chair for a two-year term; and so on. As it turned out, the most powerful, influential members of each hospital board were appointed to the system board and the hospital boards retained the less powerful members. The hospital governing boards at Trinity and Sutton Memorial would be responsible for operations, credentialing, and facilities management at their respective organizations. The powerful RRVHS board decided the hospital governing boards would no longer receive operating budgets or routine financial reports. The RRVHS board would provide financial oversight of both hospitals and control the flow of financial information. Friction soon developed between the system board and the hospital boards; they became so frustrated at one point that the two of them considered joint legal action against the system board.

The RRVHS board further decided that neither of the current hospital CEOs were capable of assuming the position of system CEO and hired an executive search firm to recruit an experienced system CEO. The RRVHS board, with powerful representatives from both hospitals, could not agree on an acceptable candidate to lead the newly merged entity. This dissension among the board members resulted in a lengthy and combative CEO search that left the new entity adrift with no management leadership for more than a year.

Curtis Tower was finally hired as RRVHS CEO. During the recruitment process, Tower made it clear that the board needed to leave the management of the new system to him, and the search committee agreed to do so. Soon after Tower assumed leadership responsibilities, it became evident the board was either unwilling or unable to stay out of the management of the new system. Once in place, Tower was directed by the RRVHS board to fire all senior administrators at both hospitals and conduct a national search to replace them. He followed this directive at the expense of losing vital corporate memory at a time when it was needed most. The corporate cultures of both organizations were visibly shaken in the process of this massive administrative turnover; organizational values were questioned by the staffs of both hospitals who were increasingly anxious in this uncertain environment.

Amid all of this uncertainty, physicians in Clay County became a major influential force. Throughout the merger process, the hospitals' two medical staffs had been relegated to the sidelines. But a new opportunity now presented itself in Richland. Physicians Partners, Inc., a proprietary corporation that purchases and operates physician practices, has begun buying physician practices in Richland. Now the RRVHS board and the two hospital boards have a common worry: what if their admitting physicians decide to admit elsewhere? A group of ten physicians who control most of the admissions, referrals, and outpatient ancillary services at both Trinity and Sutton Memorial begin approaching board members at social gatherings with an idea. These physicians had lost their ability to leverage one hospital against the other with the creation of RRVHS. Now with Physician Partners, Inc., rolling into town, the physicians have bargaining power once more. They suggest that RRVHS purchase their practices and through their personal connections to a renowned East Coast medical school, the physicians say they can arrange for the establishment of an affiliated major medical clinic in Richland that will attract national and international patients. Such a clinic will secure the success of the new merger.

RRVHS enters into what proves to be a very lucrative arrangement for the physicians involved, and news of the agreement and the planned medical school affiliated clinic disseminates rapidly throughout the medical staff community. Questions of who will control the clinic – and, more importantly, who will be allowed to practice there–are put to the RRVHS board. Dissension among the medical staff is palpable. Those physicians practicing independently give the RRVHS board an ultimatum. If plans for the clinic go ahead, they will boycott both hospitals. The RRVHS board rejects the proposed affiliated clinic. The contract physicians are angry and resentful, the independent physicians remain distrustful and hostile. Throughout these discussions, negotiations and agreements, the administrations of both hospitals have been absent.

Two years into the merger, RRVHS has yet to consolidate clinical services as recommended by the consultant's plan guiding implementation.The hospitals, four miles apart, are still duplicating all but business operations. Equally troubling is the lack of consolidation of the medical staff. The differences in medical staff organization and structure within the two hospitals have proven to be significant barriers. Medical staff officers at Trinity are elected by the general medical staff; medical staff officers at Sutton Memorial are appointed by the Sutton Memorial board. After much political maneuvering, it is agreed that consolidated medical staff officers will be elected, but this is just one more contentious issue between the two hospitals.

When the administrative offices for the system are constructed in available space at Sutton Memorial, this further increases ill-will between the hospitals. The members of the two hospital governing boards do not like one another – and, more significantly, their counterparts on the RRVHS board do not either. The governing styles of the two are in conflict. Sutton Memorial operates with a corporate approach to healthcare delivery: be innovative; operate efficiently; practice good business management. Social status is important to its members. Trinity operates more like a public institution: process-oriented; committed to care for all regardless of their ability to pay. Business operations are not its top priority and neither is the social status of its members.

But the major barriers to the successful merger of the two organizations remain the steadfast separation of all clinical services and disagreement over the allocation of capital resources for new programs and services. New clinical services to be based at one or the other hospital can never get past the planning stage. Administrative resources are spent but no program materializes in return. Frustrated and angry with the system, a high-profile group of surgeons begins plans for a physician-owned surgi-center. About this same time, amid falling patient volume and problems with accounts receivable at both hospitals, a major donor withdraws his $72 million pledge to the Cardiology program at Sutton Memorial on the grounds that his pledge was to Sutton and not to RRVHS.

Unable to consolidate clinical services and demoralized by the constant conflict and financial woes over the past three years, the RRVHS board finally agrees on something: to dissolve the merger. Within the first year following the dissolution of RRVHS, Continental Healthcare moved quickly to purchase both hospitals, that it operates as separate healthcare facilities.

Commentary

Fred L. Brown

The RRVHS seemed to have all the right things in place to deliver a new era in healthcare delivery for its community. However, what the new system possessed in potential, it lacked in execution.

I have been fortunate throughout my career to be associated with many historic and well-regarded healthcare organizations. It has been my experience that all hospitals, be they non-profit or for-profit, urban or rural, community or academic, each have a special nuance to them. But, after all is said and done, they share a common bond – a *covenant*. This covenant is to serve as stewards of valued community assets – local hospitals. This covenant is silent: that is, until change comes along. Americans expect their hospitals to be open around the clock, offer the most advanced technology, and provide a full spectrum of care and services. When that expectation is threatened, the silence is broken, and loud voices proclaim discontent and mistrust.

The healthcare merger mania of the 1990s created lots of opportunities for the silence to be broken. People were upset that their hospitals were merging – or, in some cases, even closing. Hospital mergers were touted as the right thing to do, but were viewed by the wary public as too corporate and business-like. The Richland merger illustrates these concerns very eloquently.

Several missteps occurred, and many opportunities were lost, in the Richland scenario. Drawing from my own experiences and that of many of my colleagues, I offer the following observations on what went wrong with this merger and what might have been done differently to assure its long-term success.

Fear-based

The driving force behind the merger was not one of "community betterment" but one based on *fear and power*. An outside player forced Sutton and Trinity to begin discussions. For decades, these two neighboring providers of care operated in isolation from one another; they shared no services and did not collaborate on community programs. So, from the very beginning, the foundation of the merger was on shaky ground. No community needs assessment was conducted. No base assumptions and projections were made on how the merger would best serve the more than half million residents of the community.

This was a merger of two perceived equals. The smaller, less powerful of the hospitals in the community were not taken into consideration. This was often the case in mergers in the 1990s. The Darwinian "survival of the fittest" model was too often used. This led to the impression the "Goliaths" were out to take care of their own bottom lines at the expense of the smaller, more vulnerable hospitals. It took an outside player to force these two organizations into discussions. Prior to this, the two organizations seemed to have minimal to no collaborative efforts. This fear-based merger would thus be doomed from day one.

Culture clash

If the old adage "opposites attract" holds true, it most certainly did not in this situation. Sutton and Trinity could not have been any more different. One had a strong religious affiliation and record of serving the indigent; the other had a wealthy corporate patron and served a more affluent base. Of all the warning signs against this merger, this one stands out among the crowd. How could two boards, two medical staffs, two employee groups, and two donor groups with such different historical underpinnings get along and work together?

In actuality, they might have worked great together. Since they were not historically serving the "same patient bases" *per se,* they might have found innovative ways to combine their expertise and serve the overall community. As the two most powerful and prominent healthcare facilities in the region, they had all the resources needed to make a real difference. These cultural differences could have led the way to a very effective clinical integration plan. Each organization had built-in clinical areas of expertise and areas of focus that could have respected each organization's heritage, yet served the community in a new era. Cultural integration incorporates the "human spirit issues" involved in mergers. Decades of work by physicians, board members, nurses, and volunteers must be acknowledged and this talent corralled into positive energy for the future.

Diversity

The two Richland cultures could have learned much from each other's diversity. By integrating people, programs, and policies, they could have crafted new ways to serve the 500,000 residents of Clay County. Trinity had experience in indigent care and was unionized; Sutton dealt with an older, more affluent population. The cross-pollination of these two cultures would have helped make the merger successful. The diversity of the two organizations was twofold: first, in the patients they each served and, second, in the internal "world views" within which each operated. By establishing diversity "appreciation and learning" programs in the earliest stages of the merger, employees, boards, and physicians could have learned more about their counterparts.

In healthcare, "cultural diversity" not only means race, gender, and religion, but also incorporates metropolitan and rural, urban and suburban, academic and community-based providers of care. It also encompasses types of patients served and types of staffs – nurses, therapists, physicians, board members, and community volunteers (Lerner 1997).

Diversity leads to *organizational effectiveness* in many ways (Henry and Henry 1999):

- It brings *richness of perspective and creativity* to the organization. Healthcare in particular and business in general are becoming increasingly complex. A diversity of eyes and ears widens the view on any given issue or opportunity.
- It provides heightened sensitivity to the *diversity of the organization's patient base.*
- It leads to an expanded pool of *potential workers* with varied backgrounds and skills.
- It increases the awareness and need for *effective communications skills* and techniques.
- It sensitizes organizations to their *legal, moral and social responsibility.*

With diversity on its side, Richland missed a prime opportunity to turn a perceived negative into a positive.

External forces

In addition to the overwhelming forces impacting the internal culture at Richland, external forces were also at play. Social, political, economic, and financial forces all co-exist and impact a hospital's daily life. So as the new system battled its own cultural issues, it is important to note that the outside world continued to apply daily pressures. Without internal cohesion, the new system was clearly not in a position to ensure it was proactively addressing issues such as new government regulations, managed care influences, community health status measures, and workforce shortages.

Governance

From the very beginning, these two boards could not have been more different. Although they were from the same community, their orientations were vastly opposed. The extreme micro-management role the new board assumed, despite its best of intentions, only diminished the system's success. I see two additional key issues that hampered this new board's effectiveness.

There is no question as to hospital boards' hard work and commitment. It is natural to want a strong system board that comprises as many of the former hospital board members as possible. The most practical way to handle this is to build a *governance plan* into the merger agreement. This can provide a roadmap for both interim and long-term board governance. It should outline the size of board, terms, officers, duties, rotations, and the like. During the interim phase, the new system board could have been more closely aligned with the hospital boards and have focused its efforts on more global issues that could have aided in the success of the merger. For example, the new board could have targeted one or two key projects that they could have addressed collaboratively. This might also have assisted them during the "get to know each other" phase of the merger. The newly formed health foundation, created via the $25 million garnered from Trinity's asset valuation, could also have served as a great resource for the board's community relations efforts.

Second, no physicians were added to the board. This omission has hurt and seriously compromised other mergers. This move would not just be symbolic; it would provide physicians with meaningful input into critical decisions regarding strategies and policies. In addition to physicians, other key medical professionals such as nurses make excellent board members, and should be given serious membership consideration.

If the new Richland board had found a way to balance its desire to manage operations with the need to garner key community support for the merger, it might have met with greater success. It certainly might have prevented the loss of a $72 million donation targeted at Sutton.

Leadership

By not appointing an interim CEO while the search for a permanent one took place, valuable leadership momentum was lost. An interim CEO would have given constituencies someone to follow. By not having an interim leader, there most likely would be a perception by employees that there was a lack of direction and no one was looking after their best interests. The new board also did not "inspire" trust at the employee and physician levels. An interim CEO also would have helped improve *communication* among the boards, employees, physicians, and community leaders, giving them someone to hear their concerns. Interim positions are not the most sought after jobs. However, these jobs can give administrators good and invaluable experience that can land them key leadership posts at other systems in the future.

Once Richland finally hired a CEO, they kept him on a short lease. The CEO came in with certain expectations as to his scope of duties; however, he immediately was directed to fire key administrators and this only added to the mistrust that was already pervasive throughout the new organization. This is no way to begin a "trusting" relationship between a CEO and his constituents.

Physicians

Of all the issues that Richland faced, this was the most crucial. By not involving physicians in the initial discussions, and by not appointing them to leadership posts and board positions, the discontented physicians had a stimulus to take action on their own.

In addition to board slots, Richland could have used the physicians' expertise to assist with *clinical integration.* By appointing physicians as workgroup leaders, the organization could have dealt with integration and strategic planning issues much more effectively. Increased physician input also would have helped with *employee and community relations.* People naturally look to physicians for cues as to what is happening in their hospitals.

Clinical integration

At first glance, the clinical integration component of this merger should have been one of its major accomplishments. Each hospital had very different areas of focus, and the missteps that took place throughout the merger doomed any likelihood of clinical integration success. Each hospital had specific areas of expertise and talent. But the politics of the merger made it impossible to create an atmosphere where the boards and physicians could come together to devise a rational plan.

Clinical integration is vastly simplified if governance, medical staff, and administration is complete and precedes the clinical integration process (Lerner 1997). In pursuing the clinical integration imperative, it is also vital to create a *single medical staff* for the hospitals, as well as to preserve the institutional identity and integrity, while changing the service and product mix of both organizations. If Richland could have dealt with some key administrative, board, and cultural issues in the early stages of its merger, the new system's chances for effective clinical integration would have been excellent.

Low hanging fruit

Richland's lone example of integration success appears to be that of back office operations. One of the early barometers of a merger's success often comes in the consolidations of such back office functions and through group purchasing – often termed "low-hanging fruit." The important thing to note is these cost-savings and consolidations must be put into context. How do cost-cutting, cost-saving, and quality improvement programs co-exist? And how can they thrive?

Front line involvement is key. It is crucial to establish early that the role of clinicians is to determine product acceptability, taking into consideration cost and the role of matériel services in business transactions, including the negotiation of new agreements and contracts.

Richland's lack of buy in from its key stakeholders prevented it from taking advantage of its back office operations and using the low-hanging fruit strategy as a catalyst to further integrate the two campuses – both strategically and culturally.

Employees

Communicate, communicate. This should be job one to ensure that employees at all levels are given as much information as possible during a merger transition. Employees want both the good and the bad news. They crave communication. When there is a void, that void is filled with misinformation that filters out to the community.

These key constituencies, while part of the system, cannot be reached directly by the system itself. Rather they must be reached by the individual hospitals. Patients, physicians, employees, donors, and volunteers have much greater affinity to the individual hospitals than to the new system. These audiences are still wary of the system and learn best what and why the system exists from credible and familiar sources. As the system communicates relevant milestones and demonstrates mutually strong leadership at all levels, the organization will gain credibility with these vital audiences.

It is also essential to give employees national, regional and local perspectives on what is happening in the healthcare environment, and how these issues impact their own hospitals. This gives everyone a better context about why certain decisions are being made. Town hall meetings, e-mail updates, newsletters, and videotape presentations can all be used to keep constituencies updated on system activities.

If a CEO reaches out to employees and asks for their help, they will be there for the organization. Healthcare professionals by tradition have a special calling, they have sought careers that allow them to help others. By involving employees in task forces, work groups, focus groups, and speakers' bureaus, they become empowered to help and make a difference. Considering that Richland did not include physicians at a high level, it is no surprise that employees were not more involved, and this only added to the mistrust.

The plan

By using the strategic plan provided by the outside consultants, Richland lost an opportunity to involve key constituents in important decisions. Although time-consuming, it would have been worth the effort to involve physicians, managers, and community leaders in creating a first draft strategic plan. This could have been done using outside consultants as *facilitators*. The consultants could have focused their efforts in updating the new system on industry trends, market evolutions, and other key issues, instead of penning "the plan" by themselves.

In the early stages of mergers, a strategic plan is a moving target. However, an *interim plan* with *achievable targets* provides a roadmap for a well-rounded plan that will deal with big issues such as clinical integration in the future. Examples of initiatives that an interim plan might have addressed include the consolidation of employee benefits, consolidation of one clinical service line, group purchasing savings, and creation of a new brand identity for the new system.

Baby steps

Richland, when it did act, acted much too fast. By removing the bulk of power away from the hospital boards, the new board immediately undermined these vital groups and prevented cohesion among the boards. Next, firing all senior administrators once the CEO was hired, Richland vastly added to its woes. Richland lost key "historians" who could have helped guide the new system. These administrators also had key employee and community contacts that were most likely very upset by the system's actions. By too quickly considering the physicians' "affiliation" plan, the board alienated the rest of the medical staff. By initiating a "phase one" strategic plan, the new system could have created a framework that established manageable expectations and measures of success.

In the excitement of a merger, it is just as hard to keep the wrong things from happening as it is to make the right things happen.

Symbolism

Little things mean a lot. Several missteps occurred that could have easily been addressed in this merger. First, the location of the new system offices at one of the hospitals created a less than impartial impression. Locating the offices at a neutral location, even at added expense, would probably have been for the best. The appointment of an interim CEO would also have served as a good symbolic move that things were moving forward.

Hosting various employee functions can be invaluable in symbolizing "system-ness." When the system sponsors employee days at an amusement park and athletic events, employees have an opportunity to get to know each other better. Multiple "town hall" meetings also give employees and managers a chance to be heard.

In addition, creation of a new brand identity for the system would have provided a symbolic gesture and a new focal point for the organization. Short term, the creation of a *system brand* would unite the system's products, services, facilities, and resources under a common banner that would readily identify them as being part of a new system. Over time, this helps shift awareness away from the former individual hospitals and toward services provided by the system. As parity is achieved in price and access, it is clinical excellence, customer service, and brand equity that will give a new system prime differentiation (Lerner 1997). It is however, crucial to maintain careful balance in creating a new brand identity. Just as in the Richland case, some deals go bad. So maintaining a strong individual hospital brand in conjunction with the new system identification is important, too (Sturm 1998).

Mission

The new system most likely lacked a new *mission statement.* By crafting new mission, vision, and values statements, the new system would have had a rallying and unifying focus. which would have gone a long way in helping steer the fledging system in its formative days.

"Values clarification" can also serve as the foundation for the system's first strategic plan. Explicit articulation of the organization's values, vision, and aspirations can provide a framework for making strategic choices (Coile 1998). This process can also provide the new board, physicians groups, and other key constituents with an opportunity to collaborate on common words that will lead to common actions.

Conclusion

Here are twelve basics suggestions to ensure the success of the Richland merger:
(1) Consider a *formal affiliation* prior to the full merger
(2) Include the *"smaller" hospitals* in the discussions
(3) Invest in a *pre-merger community needs and health status* analysis of region
(4) Make sure the governance structure works *strategically,* not just politically
(5) Offer *"culture change and diversity"* programs
(6) Ensure an *"interim" management team* is in place
(7) Give *physicians* key leadership roles
(8) Communicate effectively with *employees and key stakeholders*
(9) Use *consultants* for "targeted" assignments
(10) Create an initial strategic plan with *short-term targets*
(11) Give *system and hospital administrators* clear and targeted roles
(12) Establish a new *health foundation* as an example of the merger's benefit.

The failure of the Richland merger is due in great part to a breakdown in "community stewardship." The two hospitals, although different, shared a common covenant to serve the Clay County region. By not setting aside their differences and cultivating their vast resources, valuable amounts of time, money, and effort were lost. What the two hospitals feared the most happened: an outsider came into their community and took control of the local assets. However, as America continues to struggle with access to care and the uninsured, mergers can and will continue to offer market-driven solutions to local healthcare issues.

REFERENCES

Coile, R. C., Jr., 1998. *Millennium Management*. Chicago: Health Administration Press

Henry, J. and L. Henry, 1999. *Reclaiming Soul in Health Care*. Chicago: AHA Press

Lerner, W., 1997. *Anatomy of a Merger*. Chicago: Health Administration Press

Sturm, A. C., Jr., 1998. *The New Rules of Healthcare Marketing*. Chicago: Health Administration Press

14

UK review of selected cases

Robert Nicholls and Andrew Wall

Healthcare delivery systems are complex and increasingly dependent on good team-work, shared values, and accurate information. There is increasing recognition in the United Kingdom and elsewhere that, in addition to the contractual and professional duties of clinicians, the quality of management and the health of organizations have a major bearing on reducing risks to patients and providing a quality service. Although medical negligence cases are increasing in the United Kingdom, there is evidence that openness and early involvement of patients and their relatives, as well as operational staff, in handling untoward incidents is often a good defence against litigation. Similarly, in planning developments and changes in healthcare delivery, early and full involvement of key stakeholders is likely to prevent problems later.

Four of the American cases (chapters 7, 8, 10, and 11) are now reviewed by two experienced, former senior National Health Service (NHS) managers, one now working as an academic and consultant, the other chairing one of the newly created national bodies concerned with quality in the NHS. Lessons have been drawn from the cases from a UK perspective and suggestions provided as to how the cases may have been better handled.

Medical errors: Paradise Hills Medical Center

Radiation overdose is not uncommon, and this case has parallels with similar ones in the United Kingdom – notably one in the Exeter radiotherapy centre in the late 1980s (Thwaites Report 1988). Although there has been less concern in the United Kingdom with the competitive risks of a disclosure that might damage the

Management Mistakes in Healthcare, ed. Paul Hofmann and Frankie Perry. Published by Cambridge University Press. © Cambridge University Press 2005.

reputation of a hospital, other features of the case are very familiar, such as the fear of litigation and the different perspectives of medical staff members and others. Indeed it is only in the 1990s, following a number of major incidents leading to public outcry and formal inquiries (Bristol Infirmary 2001), that serious attempts were made to develop a more open culture in British hospitals aimed at learning from mistakes and reducing the risks of medical errors. Some of the specific national and local organizations and systems that have been introduced are included in the discussion of the FCH case.

What management mistakes occurred?

- While it is to the credit of Paradise Hills Medical Center management that they had in place a routine quality assurance report that allowed the board to pick up this serious medical error, it was indicative of a *medically dominated culture* that the problem was not identified sooner and a serious management error not to have reported it to the board as soon as it was discovered. Was there a culture in the Oncology department to report such incidents? Was a serious incident reporting system in place throughout the hospital? If not, these were major management shortcomings. How was a flaw in the calibration of equipment first discovered, and how was a medical physicist asked to resign without senior management knowing?

- Having recognized the problem, senior management should have taken control and acted immediately, not entering into a debate and apparently ceding the decision as to whether to notify patients of the error to the medical staff of the Oncology department, as they clearly had a *conflict of interest*.

- Given the number of patients who had received an excess radiotherapy dose and the large range of staff that had knowledge of the error, it was a bad error of judgment for management to think they could keep the matter *confidential*.

- The danger of a leak, and of both internal and external criticism, was heightened once the Ethics Committee had advised the board to inform the patients of the error. Again, it looks as if management were overly sensitive to the medical staff's views and not sufficiently aware of their *responsibilities to the patients* and the dangers of continuing to try to cover up the incident.

- When the first complaint arrived from an affected patient, the dangers of the story going public should have been recognized and the steps outlined in the next section implemented immediately rather than trying to cope with legal claims on a *one-by-one* basis.

How could the mistakes have been avoided?

- Without knowing the systems already in place at Paradise Hills Medical Center, this particular type of error and the subsequent deficient handling of mistakes might have been prevented by a good *risk management system*. This would probably have identified excessive radiation doses as a risk with relatively high occurrence in Radiotherapy departments, and with a very high significance factor in terms of danger to patients and public concern if it occurred. Machine calibration errors can be prevented by automatic alarm settings and protocols for double checks of critical settings – and, of course, regular maintenance of machines and training of operators are essential. Without knowing the reasons for the error in this case, it is not possible to be definitive about the preventative measures that might have been taken. However, the resignation of the physicist suggests that human error was a factor which called for a full investigation to discover the causes, and to identify lessons for the future.

- In view of the seriousness of the incident and the numbers of patients who might have concerns as to whether it could recur, the appropriate actions should have included:

  (1) initiating *immediate personal contact* (by phone or visit) with the patients affected
  (2) issuing a *press release*
  (3) establishing a *phone help line* to deal with inquiries from concerned patients and relatives
  (4) setting up of an *Inquiry*, possibly led by an external expert, to establish the cause of the excess doses and to make recommendations to prevent future occurrences.

- Once the Ethics Committee had advised on the need for *openness*, the Board and hospital management should have acted accordingly and implemented the steps outlined above.

- Similarly, once the first litigation case appeared, it would have been possible – and preferable – to have at least released a *reassuring statement* about the action already taken, and inviting anyone still concerned to contact the hospital.

- Given the differences of view and tensions between different factions in the Center, it would have been advisable to have some form of *review and reconciliation process* after the first case became public to consider the handling and to agree on changes for the future. It appears that there was no vehicle for allowing disagreements to be aired and relationships and confidence to be restored, so the damage to the department's reputation and functioning became long term.

Steps to be taken to avoid similar mistakes

- An *audit* should be arranged throughout the Center to ensure that the process and system requirements set out above are in place and operating effectively.

These include risk assessment, critical incident reporting, and protocols for handling serious adverse events.

- However, the most important way to prevent similar incidents in the future, and the most difficult to achieve, appears to be a *change of culture* at the Center. This would involve ensuring that patient safety and involvement in all aspects of their care was at the heart of all staff's work. It would also require a more equal balance in the relationship between disciplines and more respect from senior medical staff members for the legitimate views of others – including the board – on matters of overall patient care, ethics, and the standing of the institution.

- These are not easy matters to address and skilled *external facilitation* is likely to be required. A useful start might be to review the respective roles and authority of the key personnel in such incidents – i.e. the CEO, the Board, the Ethics Committee, the department head, the medical staff chairmen, the program directors, and the individual clinicians. This should include an examination of the difficult issue of clinical freedom *vis-à-vis* collective responsibility.

- It has taken several public scandals and a number of enquiries in the United Kingdom to start to bring about the sort of changes in attitude and relationships that this incident highlights. Since the early 1990s, a number of local and national steps have been taken to improve the quality of patient care and reduce the risks from system failures and medical mistakes. Perhaps the most important of these have included making CEOs statutorily responsible for the quality of patient services; the introduction of a formal system of clinical governance into each healthservice organization; the widespread introduction of risk management systems and risk registers; the setting up of a national Healthcare Commission; the establishment of an anonymous system of reporting errors and near misses under the auspices of the National Patient Safety Agency (DoH 2000); and an organization to help health bodies prevent and deal expeditiously with problems arising with doctors and dentists – the National Clinical Assessment Authority (DoH 2001). Many of these initiatives have been led by the Government's Chief Medical Officer, Professor Sir Liam Donaldson, who is personally committed to raising the quality of patient care (DoH 2003a).

Although there is much still to be achieved, the culture in the NHS is gradually changing from being closed and defensive to being more open and willing to learn from mistakes, and from retrospective attempts to identify blame to better anticipation of risks and an emphasis on prevention. This is not to say that incidents such as the one described in this case no longer arise; the important thing is to have robust systems in place to handle them properly, and in the public interest, when they do.

Nursing Shortage: Metropolitan Community Hospital

The problems at Metropolitan Community Hospital (MCH) serve as a useful warning to developing situations in the United Kingdom's NHS. Competition between hospitals was introduced by the 1990 National Health Service and Community Care Act. It was the belief of the then Conservative government that competition would improve efficiency and flush out poor clinical practice. Fourteen years later, the arguments still rage. Currently, the Labour government wishes to experiment with the introduction of what they have called Foundation Hospitals that, it claims, will give more autonomy to those hospitals, which are already perceived – using selected criteria – to be successful. Those who oppose this policy point out that it may increase local competition not so much for patients, because there is not the range of choices available to many US populations, but for staff. In responding to this criticism, the government points to another national policy document *Agenda for Change* (DoH 2003b), that specifically limits opportunities for hospitals to "poach" each other's staff by means of pay differentials.

That these two policy initiatives are potentially incompatible is, critics say, a characteristic of the current government's lack of "joined-up thinking." On the one hand, local initiatives are encouraged while, on the other, compliance with nation-wide policies is required. Those same critics are likely to be critical of too much local autonomy, using situations such as that at MCH to justify their concerns.

However, the problems facing MCH potentially face all organizations, whatever the context. Here we have a "sick" organization, characterized by conflict, lack of trust, lack of respect, and an inability to prioritize.

How might a UK chief executive approach the problem?

Diagnosis

It is clear that the organization is *dysfunctional*. The first step must be to involve all the staff and the board in accepting the nature of the problems. All staff are potential losers if the present situation continues. The use of an outside consultant is essential in this situation so that diagnosis and prescription are not compromised by existing affiliations and loyalties. Such a consultant would be expected to propose a program of multi-disciplinary group meetings where there is an understanding that all participants are equal and consequently all views have potential value, irrespective of profession, rank, or grade. Once the problems are accepted as having implications for everyone, the possibility of finding remedies becomes more likely.

Potential solutions

One of the most obvious issues is whether Jane should move on. She has been in post twelve years and her relationships have become somewhat ritualized. Most organizations would be tempted to move her on. But before making this choice, it is worth considering the alternative. While it may be true that Jane has been too long in her job to alter her perception of the problems – and, more particularly, her relationships both with her own staff and the doctors – it is not necessarily a good thing to remove her. This will be seen as a symbolic act but will not of itself lead to fundamental change. Indeed, it will encapsulate the problem as being one of a single personality. In fact, as we have seen, the difficulties are endemic. Far more powerful would be for Jane to be able to change, to demonstrate that a new way of approaching issues can lead to a healthier situation. She will have strengths as well as weaknesses: for example, she will be able to provide some degree of corporate memory. If she is helped to approach aspects of her job in a new way, she will be a powerful exemplar of the changes that are needed.

There are clearly examples within the organization of successful departments. Too simplistic a use of these departments as beacons may merely cause resentment elsewhere, but it is possible that there are *change agents* from among their staff who could help others more subtly to work through partnership issues.

It is customary in such a situation to spend time on developing a new *mission statement*. Care needs to be taken here. Such statements habitually end up as platitudinous and are perceived by staff and patients alike with some degree of cynicism. Therefore, the value is in discussing what *principles* should support a mission statement, rather than the end result. In this way, the overall values of the organization can be explored to see to what extent there can be common ground.

Whereas the problem is primarily internal, external issues such as competition from other providers and nursing accommodation issues should not be ignored. Practically speaking, would some help with accommodation costs help nurses, particularly those from overseas? Although commercially risky, is it worth having discussions with the other providers to limit the stranglehold of the agencies, as all are at risk? The United Kingdom is facing this dilemma, where agencies threaten to absorb the large sums of extra money awarded to the NHS by government, with little tangible improvement in the quality of care.

Finally, enlisting community leaders in defining the health needs of the total community may help to ensure that MCH is seen more as a service than a commercial enterprise.

Inept strategic planning: Southwestern Regional Healthcare System

In the United Kingdom until the 1960s, about 40% of deliveries took place out of hospital, mostly in the mother's own home. The Cranbrook Report (MoH 1959) reviewed existing practice and in particular noted the number of perinatal (stillbirths and deaths within one week of live births) and maternal deaths. Both rates were considered unsatisfactory. The result was to increase the expert supervision of mothers in both the pre-natal period and at the point of delivery. As a result, about 98% of births now take place in hospital, although not all of these will be in a central acute unit.

There has been a backlash from mothers who feel that the normal process of giving birth has been unduly medicalized. A Department of Health policy document *Changing Childbirth* (1993) recommended a more sensitive approach, recognizing that as at least a third of all births have no complications the mother should have the right of choice in deciding where to have her baby. Despite this, there has been only a slow change in practice, mostly by transferring the primary clinical responsibility of low-risk mothers to midwives away from increasingly reluctant general practitioners. This change, where it has happened, does not seem to have resulted in any increased risk to mother or baby.

In comparison with the United States, it is unusual for any mother to be more than twenty-five miles from an acute unit, so that unforeseen complications during birth can result in an immediate transfer or a visit from the obstetric "flying squad" that will attend the mother and supervise transfer if necessary. It would be unusual to use a helicopter in such cases.

The problem's at the Southwestern Regional Healthcare System (SRHS) need to be examined from four perspectives: medical, economic, strategic, and user.

Medical

The number of births in LaPaz, even among a young population, is relatively small. It is doubtful that running a satellite service is a good use of SRHS' medical expertise. Such expertise would be more effectively utilized by setting up an *outreach educational program* keeping the primary care staff, doctors and midwives, up to date.

The possibility of a 'domino' scheme could be explored whereby mothers are admitted for delivery only, being discharged the same day if all is well. This would ensure that deliveries took place in an optimum setting without underly over-medicalizing the event.

Economic

An outreach service can be managed only at a relatively high cost. The numbers are small, the workload slight. The opening of additional beds is wasteful as it is likely that a three-bed unit in the existing hospital would be enough to meet need.

Strategic

What business is SRHS in? It appears that its strengths are in specialist and tertiary care so why get involved in obstetrics, particularly as this is a specialty with high risk of litigation? It might be considered that once mothers have become involved with SRHS' services they will thereafter choose SRHS for subsequent pediatric and other care, but given the small numbers, this attempt to generate market loyalty seems unlikely to bring much return.

User

Many mothers resent the medicalization of childbirth. On the other hand, they may be quick to allocate blame if something goes wrong. A balance must therefore be found. Pre- and post-natal care needs the continuity which only local staff can provide. Mothers are more likely to trust staff they know rather than visiting staff they do not.

Conclusion

If SRHS still wishes to be involved in this community – and it must be questioned whether it is worth their while to be so – then its best intervention would be to help educate the clinical staff to ensure high standards of obstetric practice rather than attempt to run a satellite service at high cost.

Public relations crisis: The George C. Fremont Community Hospital

While this case has some parallels to the medical errors case (chapter 7) in that, in part, it concerns the communications strategy following a serious equipment failure with a tragic outcome, in some ways it appears more serious, as there seems to have been a deliberate attempt at a cover-up by the CEO. Again it has features that will be familiar to UK readers, recalling similar efforts to cover up bad news which were prevalent in the early 1990s. The development of a more transparent and professional approach to handling communications and public relations over the last few years means that this sort of case is less likely to occur now in an NHS institution.

Management mistakes

- Apart from possible system failures that led to the equipment malfunction, once the incident had been reported, it would have better to *suspend*, not discharge, the staff involved in order that events leading to the tragedy could be fully established before blame was apportioned and resentment amongst key staff created.
- It was a bad error of judgment to think that such an event could be kept *confidential* when so many people were aware of, and upset by, the tragedy. It meant that those most closely involved were not brought in to: (1) establish the causes; (2) ensure that lessons were identified to prevent a recurrence; and (3) share this information with other hospitals and the equipment manufacturers.

- Ignoring the professional advice of his Director of Media Relations was clearly a bad error as was the decision to avoid reporting it to the board. In the current climate in the United Kingdom, these failures would almost certainly have led to the termination of the CEO's contract.

How could mistakes been avoided?

- There should have been early recognition of the likelihood that the seriousness of the incident would become *public*.
- The initiative could have been seized by establishing the causes of the equipment failure and *communicating fully* with the relatives (accepting responsibility on behalf of the hospital) and the local media.
- A full *internal or external investigation* should have occurred before apportioning blame and taking disciplinary action.
- The *staff of the department* should have been involved in the inquiry to determine whether any other patients could be at risk from a similar fault and to take appropriate preventative steps – including reporting to the manufacturers.

Steps to avoid a recurrence

- The absence of *clear protocols* for handling major clinical incidents and the subsequent communications issues seem to lie at the heart of the management failures in this case. Protocols should be developed and approved by the Board.
- There appears to be a need to create a climate of *openness and trust* at the most senior levels in the organization, and some specific training or executive coaching will be needed for the CEO, if he retains his post.
- As with the medical errors case (chapter 7), in the United Kingdom there are now national systems for reporting such incidents to both the Patient Safety Agency and to the Medical Devices Agency. Where necessary, these agencies can issue a general alert to hospitals using the same type of equipment. Most NHS boards now employ or retain public relations specialists who would be expected to handle the communications aspects of such a case.
- Locally, the *statutory duty* on the Chief Executive of NHS Trusts to promote the quality of services and the development of clinical governance systems has done a great deal to ensure that appropriate processes are in place to prevent or deal with such incidents.

REFERENCES

Bristol Infirmary, 2001. *The Inquiry into the Management of the Care of Children Receiving Complex Heart Surgery at the Bristol Royal Infirmary*. The Bristol Infirmary Inquiry, July

DoH, 2000. *An Organisation with a Memory*. London: Department of Health, June

2001. *Assuring the Quality of Medical Practice – Implementing Supporting Doctors, Protecting Patients*. London: Department of Health, January

2003a. *Annual Report of the Chief Medical Officer 2002*. London: Department of Health, July

2003b. *Agenda for Change*. London: HMSO

DoH Expert Maternity Group, 1993. *Changing Childbirth* (Cumberlege Report). London: HMSO

MoH, 1959. *Report of the Maternity Services Committee* (Cranbrook Report). London: HMSO

Thwaites Report, 1988. The *Thwaites Report on the Exeter Inquiry*. London: HMSO

15

Lessons learned: insights and admonitions

Paul B. Hofmann and Frankie Perry

The influence of ego and personal values on organizational culture

As emphasized in our preface and chapter 1, acknowledging and examining mistakes in healthcare management is not a common activity. Nonetheless, it is indisputable that significant mistakes have occurred, and some errors are inevitable. Unfortunately, while clinical errors occur with greater frequency than we are comfortable in admitting, the number and magnitude of management mistakes is even less well acknowledged. The aggregate economic and non-economic costs are incalculable. Moreover, because these mistakes occur in hospitals and other healthcare settings, patients, families, and communities are adversely affected, not just employees, physicians, executives, and board members. US Representative Pete Stark has said that healthcare executives should be held to a higher standard of ethics and compliance than their counterparts at non-healthcare companies, "because mistakes and a cavalier attitude can cause serious harm or even death. At least nobody died at Enron. We're seeing a culture of apathy in health care that's too bad" (Taylor 2003).

Some executives have large egos, and many do not invite – or, in certain cases, even permit – constructive criticism of their decisions. Conventional wisdom suggests that the more senior the executive, the less likely that person will be informed of mistakes. Regrettably, management hubris can contribute to professional hypocrisy. Executives find ways to excuse or defend their mistakes when they would never condone such behavior by others. Fear of criticism from influential stakeholders (managers, board members, physicians, employees, or the media) can

Management Mistakes in Healthcare, ed. Paul Hofmann and Frankie Perry. Published by Cambridge University Press. © Cambridge University Press 2005.

inhibit timely disclosure, but delay is both unwise and counterproductive. Not disclosing or aggressively confronting a mistake out of timidity or embarrassment compounds the error. In these situations, pain deferred is not pain avoided. Indeed, it is likely that the pain will be much greater.

Even more disturbing are attempts to cover-up mistakes. As has been observed with medical errors, "It is far more damaging to conceal than reveal" (Blustein, Post, and Dubler 2002). Conscientious executives will always defend a position that they are convinced is right, but it takes a higher degree of integrity to admit and accept responsibility promptly when they are wrong. Such candor remains too rare, and the reasons are self-evident. Relevant here is John F. Kennedy's comment following the disastrous Bay of Pigs invasion: "Success has a thousand fathers; failure is an orphan."

Admitting mistakes to oneself is the first step in disclosure. Rationalizing or hiding small mistakes can result in larger mistakes, so both the individual and the organization will benefit if more emphasis is placed on acknowledging errors, rather than trying to justify or conceal them. Disclosing inconvenient truths is difficult and unpleasant, but an executive who demonstrates a tendency to repress bad news is promoting an unhealthy organizational culture, one in which the likelihood of implementing timely corrective measures is severely compromised. Personal as well as institutional integrity and credibility are at stake (Hofmann 2003). Consequently, the optimal culture will encourage a focus on:

- *Disclosing* errors, not ignoring or concealing them
- Analyzing the *reasons* for mistakes, not rationalizing their occurrence
- Searching for *solutions*, not embarrassing individuals
- Developing and implementing *effective preventive measures*, not presuming the problem was an isolated incident
- Stimulating a *learning environment* that finds value in mistakes, not creating a punitive atmosphere that discourages innovative behavior.

The inextricable link between ethical challenges and management errors

Not surprisingly, as financial and non-financial pressures on healthcare institutions intensify, moral lapses in judgment will increase. And, as executives encounter more ethical challenges, there is a higher probability that serious errors will be made. Such challenges include:

- Allocating resources fairly
- Implementing appropriate cost containment initiatives
- Preserving confidentiality of information
- Safeguarding against abusive and fraudulent billing practices

- Resolving and preventing conflicts of interest
- Balancing organizational and community needs
- Assuring proper physician payment arrangements
- Dealing with incompetent or marginally competent employees and physicians.

These issues are not new, but when executives fail to take action or exercise poor judgment, the consequences can be devastating – impacting patients, families, staff, and entire communities.

In the preface to their 1999 landmark report, *To Err Is Human: Building a Safer Health System* (Institute of Medicine) the authors, who called attention to the 44,000–98,000 Americans dying each year in hospitals as a result of clinical errors, said: "Human beings, in all lines of work, make errors. Errors can be prevented by designing systems that make it hard for people to do the wrong thing and easy for people to do the right thing . . . As health care and the system that delivers it become more complex, the opportunities for errors abound". Although this report concentrated on clinical mistakes affecting patient care, many of the underlying observations and recommendations are directly relevant to addressing management mistakes, such as:

- Improving decision-making processes
- Disclosing errors
- Evaluating causes
- Implementing preventive measures
- Eliminating a culture of blame.

Key issues addressed in the book

Although it is impractical to comment on all the major issues covered by the contributing authors, there are a number that deserve special attention. Reviewing the earlier chapters with a focus on salient points, commonalities, and recommendations for managing mistakes will be helpful.

Valuable lessons can be learned from one's mistakes and from the mistakes of others. Unfortunately, management mistakes are not always easy to recognize. They may be acts of omission as well as commission, *and* some will be unavoidable. The inevitability of management mistakes is lamentable, but becoming paralyzed by the fear of making a management mistake can be much worse. Disclosing management mistakes and developing appropriate coping strategies is essential to improving management performance.

In chapter 1, Hofmann looks at what happens to professionals when a mistake is made. *Defining an executive error* is not always easy; much depends on the circumstances, and from whose perspective the circumstances are being viewed. Compared to medicine, defining management mistakes may be more difficult because standards of performance are not as clear. Furthermore, there is an "understandable resistance" on the part of an executive to acknowledge mistakes. Fears of reprimand, job loss, legal repercussions, and humiliation constitute strong motives for silence. An executive may rationalize mistakes made in order to preserve self-esteem. And in fact, there may be some doubt that a mistake actually occurred: there are cases where things just "don't work out." A working definition of a mistake helps to establish its parameters – "making a decision to act or not act without thoroughly assessing known evidence and incorporating stakeholders' perspectives when the action or inaction (a) places patients, staff, the organization, and/or the community at risk, or (b) is costly to implement, or (c) costly to change." Three categories of mistakes are identified here:

(1) Negligence
(2) Decisions or non-decisions that produce bad outcomes not intended
(3) Mistakes that do not produce bad outcomes.

Intentional wrongdoing is excluded from the discussions. These mistakes can be attributed to a range of motives, including anger, greed, and indifference.

Organizational culture has a powerful influence on whether management mistakes are recognized and analyzed. An organization with a zero tolerance for mistakes is simply being unrealistic. Rather, the organizations should strive to be "learning organizations [where] mistakes [can] also be viewed as opportunities for promoting individual growth and development." The context for healthcare management mistakes is complex and full of a "host of issues . . . that . . . make the difficulties seem overwhelming." Contributing to these challenges is the power and influence of the medical staff. Physicians occasionally intimidate patients, families, and staff. Unlike their corporate counterparts, healthcare managers have long struggled with the "dual lines of authority" that exist in healthcare delivery. Likewise, improper exercise of authority in management can "repress legitimate questioning" of those in power. Generally, mistakes should be disclosed to those most affected by them and to those in authority. Policies on disclosure should be developed ahead of time and in advance of a crisis. Admitting, analyzing, and disclosing errors is a mark of "management maturity." Coping with one's mistakes and their disclosure requires a level of humility, the acceptance of one's fallibility, and compassion toward oneself. Improving management performance requires that "systems are implemented to prevent, discourage, detect, and address mistakes." Appropriate attention to management mistakes also requires "a board that is deliberative, well informed and with a relationship with the CEO based on mutual trust and respect." Joyce Godwin writes more about the responsibilities of governance in chapter 12(p.180).

In chapter 2, John Worthley suggests that to benefit from our mistakes and the mistakes of others, we must examine the *context* in which management mistakes occur. He distinguishes eight major dimensions to be explored: legal, organizational, financial, political, professional, ethical, social, and psychological. The legal dimension is visible and directive; Worthley describes the panoply of laws, rules, regulations, and procedures that govern healthcare operations as useful in helping the healthcare manager to avoid making mistakes.

When discussing the *organizational context* in which mistakes occur, Worthley reminds us that mistakes are usually the result of both individuals and the environment in which they occur. Both formal and informal organizational realities facilitate or minimize mistakes within an organization, and the degree of consistency between the two greatly influences the occurrence of mistakes, their disclosure, and how they are managed. He indicates that the most frequent mistakes involve cover-ups of incidents, falsifying reports, deceiving clients, withholding information, and cutting corners. Financial fears and pressures play a significant role in the occurrence of management mistakes, especially when reward systems are tied to financial performance. Recent corporate scandals provide solid evidence for this observation.

Worthley advises that attention be paid to the political dimension affecting management mistakes. He notes that politics are "a healthy and normal reality of everyday human life, including organizational life" and have very real influence on what transpires within organizations.

While most organizations have ethical mechanisms in place to guide staff conduct, Worthley notes that the ethical dimension is sometimes overlooked when economic considerations take precedent. Issues such as patient's rights and quality of care, for example, may get short shrift in the face of economic concerns.

The social and psychological dimensions are no less important. For example, the notion that "if everyone does it, it must be acceptable" has great influence on the activities of some managers. In many cases, the relentless drive for corporate or personal success leads managers to justify their mistakes. Worthley offers the "conscious quest of a bias for 'diversity of thought and ideas' at corporate, group, and individual levels within an organization" as the antidote for these pressures.

Worthley provides the reader with a valuable analysis of the organizational context within which management mistakes occur. It explores both the formal and informal realities of an organization that contribute to mistakes, and the way they are handled. His matrix (Table 2.1, p.31) suggests that the formal and informal realities each consist of a corporate, group, and individual dimension, all of which interact and impact one another. Power is one element of the informal realities within an organization that deserves further discussion here. In his book

The Ethics of the Ordinary in Healthcare (1997), Worthley provides a primer for six sources of professional power. They are as follows:

(1) *Coercive* power – subordinates treat supervisors with deference and compliance out of fear of reprisal

(2) *Connective* power – the one in power is needed for access so she is given power and compliance with her whims in order to gain favor or avoid disfavor

(3) *Presumed expertise* – the one in power is perceived to have expertise or knowledge that is needed so deference is paid

(4) *Information* – the one in power has information or access to information that is needed so deference is paid

(5) *Rewards* – it is believed that the one in power will bestow rewards if deference is paid

(6) *Legitimacy* – the one in authority is granted power by virtue of her position (Worthley 1997:63–64).

Yet another source of power is "paternalistic power," where subordinates seek the approval of the "parent" authority and want nothing more than to please the supervisor (Perry 2001). Power also lies in the rituals and symbols that structure and influence human interactions. Berger and Luckmann (1967) posit the theory that all reality is socially constructed by the interactions of the participants and that rituals and symbols designate where the power exists in each interaction. It can be argued that the power or perceived power within corporate, group, and individual interactions may be the singularly most influential element in determining whether management mistakes are made – and, if made, whether they are recognized and/or disclosed.

In chapter 3, Wanda Jones begins by providing the reader with her shorthand definition of a mistake: "A decision that leads to negative consequences, which could have been avoided, made by an individual in a position of responsibility or by a governing board on the advice of that person, or by any other person." "It *is* rectitude," she says, "acting from the basis of principle and character, that separates the value-free bureaucrat from the leader."

Jones recognizes the complexity of decision-making within healthcare management, and allows that many management decisions are arrived at through consensus. In spite of this, she maintains that those in authority remain accountable for these decisions. Furthermore, Jones makes it clear that CEOs and healthcare managers have accountability in the delivery of clinical services by:

(1) Seeing that the right programs are developed in response to community need

(2) Making sure these programs remain scientifically current

(3) Providing adequate staffing

(4) Ensuring that the medical staff members practice the highest standards of care

(5) Supplying needed resources.

This is an important point because there are those who attempt to distinguish between *management* and *clinical* decisions and deny management accountability in clinical affairs, as in the Tenet Healthcare case discussed in chapter 6. Jones also is clear on the responsibility of healthcare management to develop initiatives in response to community health needs – and, indeed, to advocate for community health. She views a failure to act in this regard as a management mistake.

Jones provides an in-depth analysis of the various classifications of mistakes followed by an analysis of the main ways that mistakes are discovered, such as regularly reviewing and evaluating past decisions, direct observation, audits, issues raised by physicians, staff or board, litigation, etc. Jones then offers suggestions for "creating a cultural climate in which all managers are able to prevent, admit and act on mistakes" and follows up with a few personal rules of behavior which bear repeating here:

(1) Tell the truth consistently
(2) Educate board members so they trust what you say and they know that you will do what you say
(3) Get to know physicians and staff so they know your inner character
(4) Celebrate the positive things people do
(5) Discuss ethical decision-making so people know what you expect
(6) Create a corporate culture that shares an understanding of how the organization works
(7) Measure, report and scrutinize decision-making results
(8) Back up your managers
(9) Nurture your inner peace
(10) Stay committed to the best interests of patients and community.

In summary, Jones wisely reminds us that a significant reason for dealing carefully with mistakes is the *life-affecting nature* of healthcare. While physicians have a long-standing tradition of assessing clinical performance, managers have not always emulated their clinical colleagues by making an objective evaluation of management performance. Failure to recognize that management decisions can impact clinical services and may compromise patient care can have devastating results.

In chapter 4, Carol Bayley suggests that much of what has been learned in the field of medical errors can be effectively translated into the discipline of management. She begins by emphasizing that in both medical and management mistakes, the *organizational culture* plays a significant role. She stresses the need for organizations to move from a "blame and shame" culture to a "culture of organizational learning" that uses errors to analyze and re-design the systems and structures that produced them. Like Wanda Jones in chapter 3, Bayley, too, holds managers accountable for patient care issues: "Prospective responsibility for patient safety . . . resides in the collective that comprises not only direct care providers but managers and administrators as well, since their decisions about staffing, equipment, and policies contribute to or prevent potential errors." Bayley proposes that organizational "culture is grown deliberately, through the decisions that managers and employees make, and by accident, by what is allowed . . . and what flows from strong personalities." She suggests that when a medical error occurs, management has proof that something went wrong in the system and now has an opportunity to make system or process changes that will prevent similar errors from occurring in the future. Thus, management errors and medical errors are intertwined. In summary, Bayley notes that an organizational culture of *trust and transparency*, cultivated by management, will allow an organization to learn and to grow from mistakes of any kind. Without such a culture, there can be no improvement in quality or safety.

In chapter 5, John Russell and Benn Greenspan acknowledge the inevitability of management mistakes, and offer suggestions to avoid them and to minimize their impact when they occur. They caution that if managers are appropriately decisive, they will make mistakes. Further, if managers are to be effective, they must be prepared to take risks, make decisions, incur mistakes, and learn from the experience. The key here is to "celebrate and learn from mistakes." Russell and Greenspan indicate that the biggest mistake that managers consistently make is not recognizing that they have the wrong person in a key position and failing to do anything about it. Hiring the right person to do the job can be a major challenge, but it is important in minimizing management mistakes. Other recommendations offered for avoiding and correcting management errors include:

(1) Making sure our actions can withstand public scrutiny
(2) Pursuing objectivity in correcting mistakes and changing strategy
(3) Recognizing poor communication as a reason for failure.

Among Russell and Greenspan's recommendations for preventing management mistakes include:

(1) Using case studies to learn about management mistakes
(2) Maintaining public trust by strengthening governance and accountability
(3) Developing a management problem-solving methodology
(4) Making reduction of medical *and* management errors a top priority
(5) Appreciating timing as a critical factor in management decisions
(6) Knowing your core business and sticking to it
(7) Combining sound management and social vision
(8) Supplementing evidence-based medicine with evidence-based management.

Emily Friedman adroitly tackles the issue of accountability in chapter 6. She notes that accountability rests with the person who commits the error as well as the person on whose watch the error is committed. The higher one resides in the organizational hierarchy, the greater the level of accountability: accountability and consequences go hand in hand.

Friedman reminds readers that healthcare delivery is different from the corporate world because people trust their lives to the system. They frequently have no choice in selecting their providers, and little knowledge upon which to judge their care. Nonetheless, they are highly intolerant of errors. Society has offered few rewards for admitting one's errors and great rewards for concealing them; consequently, members of society tend to blame someone else or uncontrollable circumstances for their own blunders. The "no-fault society" we currently inhabit means that there are often little or no consequences for those who do own up to their mistakes or whose mistakes are discovered by others.

Friedman believes, however, a shift may be occurring. Recent corporate scandals have prompted new regulations and laws that promise to bring more account-ability to the corporate world and to the healthcare industry. Friedman offers a number of very sound reasons for having accountable organizations:

(1) Wrongdoing will always be discovered and punished
(2) Healthcare organizations depend on the good will of the community
(3) Being perceived as trustworthy has a market advantage
(4) A reputation for integrity is a bonus in the employment market
(5) Patients and payers are pushing for higher quality and reliability
(6) Not being accountable is career-limiting behavior
(7) Being true to a moral code leads to a happier life and a happier organization.

She also suggests several means by which a healthcare executive can establish accountability for herself and within her sphere of influence:

(1) Know who you hire
(2) Make integrity the priority
(3) Have oversight of executive performance and a means of reporting failure
(4) Have a culture where there is no fear in reporting an error, a process for limiting harm, investigating what happened, and preventing future occurrences
(5) Have a culture that encourages facing consequences
(6) Have a chain of accountability instead of a "search for villains."

Finally, Friedman suggests that accountable leadership is necessary, but will not be sustainable if it does not have an *accountable organization* to lead. She provides the reader with steps that can be taken to make the organization an accountable entity. In summary, Friedman notes that accountability has been elusive, but it is the "heart and soul of healthcare" and "with it, . . . organizations can weather any storm." Without it, the consequences can be devastating.

Assessment of cases, commentaries, and common themes

Having reviewed the highlights of chapters 1–6, let us now take a look at the seven cases that followed and examine their relationship to these chapters. Each case was drawn from a real set of events in a healthcare organization.

Paradise Hills Medical Center, (chapter 7) and the George C. Fremont Community Hospital (chapter 11) are both cases that center around medical errors and management's responsibility both before and after the medical errors occurred. Throughout chapters 1–6, author after author stressed management's responsibility and accountability for clinical services. Russell and Greenspan in chapter 5 make it clear when they say: "The quality of our clinical product is our first responsibility." Bayley in chapter 4 proposes that when a medical error occurs, it signifies a *system failure* and provides an opportunity for management to change systems or processes to prevent future errors. Friedman in chapter 6 provides the reader with a recent Tenet case that clearly illustrates management accountability for clinical services. When cardiac surgeons at a Tenet Healthcare hospital were accused of performing unnecessary and risky surgery on patients, a Tenet spokesperson said that "this is an investigation of doctors, not the hospital or Tenet." It was alleged, however, that the hospital executives "looked the other way" because of the substantial revenue being generated by these surgeons. Despite its previous claims that it had nothing to do with the situation, Tenet agreed to pay $54 million in fines to the federal government and the state of California.

In the Paradise Hills Medical Center and the George C. Fremont Community Hospital cases (chapters 7 and 11), not only did management deny accountability for medical errors, they attempted to conceal them from the patients, the families, and the public. In chapter 2, Worthley reminds us that one of the most frequently made management mistakes is the cover-up of an unfortunate incident. Later in that same chapter, he notes that issues such as patient rights are sometimes overlooked out of consideration for economic issues. That observation certainly seems relevant in these two cases. In chapter 1, Hofmann recommends that mistakes, first and foremost, should be disclosed to those *most affected* by them. In these two cases, that would most certainly be the patients and their families. A fundamental issue in these two cases is that of truth telling. Can there be any public trust in these two organizations once the truth comes out?

Russell and Greenspan in chapter 5 caution that organizations should make certain that their actions can withstand public scrutiny. In the Paradise Hills Medical Center case, hospital leadership deferred to the medical staff and abdicated their responsibility in clinical affairs. Unfortunately, this is not all that uncommon. When you have interaction of multiple professionals with conflicting goals, the stage is set for mistakes to occur. In Ruth Rothstein's commentary following the George C. Fremont Community Hospital case, she cites a similar incident at her organization where the medical staff and management worked together to disclose the medical error to the patient and family, and negative consequences to the hospital were averted as a result. Emily Friedman in chapter 6 emphasizes that those who seek healthcare services have no choice because they cannot heal themselves. They have little or no information with which to judge their care. They simply must trust the system and the professionals who care for them. When that trust is violated, it can never be fully restored.

Perhaps the predominant theme throughout the chapters and the cases that followed is the significant role that *organizational culture* plays in acknowledging and addressing management mistakes. Every author has identified the need for a "learning organization," one that is transparent in all of its dealings and one that has replaced the "blame and shame" culture with one where mistakes are used as opportunities to improve services. There is no doubt that leadership plays a critical role in the cultivating and nurturing of an organizational culture where management mistakes can be admitted, investigated, and used for good. Healthcare managers at every level of the organization, however, must not lose sight of their responsibility for the culture within their sphere of influence. Throughout this work, the reader is provided with useful ideas for developing such a learning organization. Wanda Jones' practical suggestions in chapter 3 remind us that developing a positive organizational culture is a fundamental management responsibility and not an optional obligation. She suggests placing more discipline and objectivity into the planning and evaluation of decisions, searching for mistakes in the form of obsolescence, incompetence, or inappropriateness, and supplying managers with modern tools that allow oversight and early detection of problems. One of the most often-mentioned tools in earlier chapters was *root-cause analysis*. Many of the contributing authors propose the use of this JCAHO recommended tool to ferret out the root cause of "sentinel events" and the management mistakes that often accompany them.

The governance of an organization is not exempt from responsibility for the culture of the organization and the culture that permeates the governance structure itself. The governing boards at Southwestern Regional Healthcare System (chapter 10), Pleasant Valley Regional Health System (chapter 12) and Sutton Memorial Hospital (chapter 13), operated in a culture of "arrogance" which they then imposed upon the organizations for which they had fiduciary responsibility. This organizational arrogance resulted in a satellite hospital failure, missed opportunities in managed care, and a failed merger, respectively. These failures were costly in terms of dollars, time, and human capital. Management responsibility in these cases for fair and honest evaluation of resources allocation based on patient and community need cannot be overlooked: it is a matter of public trust. The CEOs in these organizations bear enormous responsibility for these failures and for their omission to deal capably with ineffective, inappropriate governing boards. Jones makes it clear in chapter 3 that the CEO has a responsibility to remedy an obsolete governance system; Joyce A. Godwin, in her commentary on chapter 12, skillfully describes management's role in governance transformation and redesign.

Throughout chapters 1–6 and the cases that follow, there is an additional common denominator that is a major contributing factor in the conflicts, problems, and management mistakes that are made – the *relationship of people and their different values*, along with the *special interests* and *goals* that each person brings to the workplace. Healthcare executives often find the management of people, as opposed to other resources, to be the most difficult part of their jobs. Diversity of the workforce, professional loyalties and differences, and time pressures compound this task.

Paradise Hills Medical Center (chapter 7) is a vivid example of conflicting goals and values among professional disciplines. Metropolitan Community Hospital (chapter 8) is fraught with interpersonal conflicts between nursing superiors and subordinates, between American and foreign nurses and between nurses and physicians. These conflicts underlie the nursing shortage crisis that the hospital is experiencing. Failing to deal with these conflicts by conducting a root-cause analysis of the nursing shortage and implementing immediate remedial steps is an indefensible management failure.

The IT setback at Heartland Healthcare System (chapter 9) is "a . . . 'crisis of confidence' in the . . . leadership capabilities . . . at the top," according to Mark Neaman. How did the well-intended goal of developing a state-of-the art IT system turn into such a crisis? Failure to hire the right people, failure to diagnose the underlying organizational psychology, failure to empower operations staff, and failure to anticipate and prevent the intra-staff warfare that ensued were all failures to manage people appropriately.

Staffing, recruitment, retention, and evaluation of employee performance are critical management functions and must be given necessary attention. It is the employees that drive an organization, create the culture, and determine whether the organization succeeds or fails. Consequently, *team building* is important in the achievement of organizational goals that often cross over departmental boundaries. Management must promote teamwork, as it integrates the efforts of staff to achieve organizational goals. Failure to work effectively with unions, to compassionately and fairly manage workforce reduction, and to foster open and honest communication with employees, can create an organizational climate of *distrust and negativity* that promises disaster.

Value of a UK perspective

The UK perspective on acknowledging and addressing management errors provides valuable insights for healthcare managers, regardless of their country of residence and employment. We learn that healthcare organizations throughout the world have more in common than not. We all have patients presenting for care; professionals with differing values and goals; acute staffing needs; and an interest in preserving the public trust, regardless of how different our "publics" may be. It is interesting to note that healthcare organizations in the United Kingdom, with its NHS, do not concern themselves with competition for patients, but they do compete vigorously for staff, so much so that there is a national policy that limits "poaching" each other's staff by means of pay differentials.

Medical errors are not uncommon in the United Kingdom and while there is less concern about the competitive risks of disclosure, there remains the fear of litigation and public scorn. Following a number of major incidents and the subsequent public outcry, there have been efforts to develop a more open culture in British hospitals that learns from mistakes, not unlike similar efforts in the United States. Notable local and national changes include policies that mandate that CEOs be responsible for the quality of patient services. Risk management systems have also been implemented in Britain in an attempt to mitigate litigation. As in America, management must be cautious to make appropriate decisions without undue influence of legal counsel; fear of litigation may lead to improper decisions that are not always in the best interests of patients.

Karen Ignagni (2003), President and CEO of the American Association of Health Plans, has noted that:

Transparency is essential . . . Adverse events must be systematically reported and clinicians and researchers must be able to analyze them thoroughly, from underlying causes to ultimate consequences. This is simply not going to happen on a consistent or reliable basis unless a climate can be created in which individuals and institutions can acknowledge honest errors without fearing that doing so could invite retribution on a scale that may be wildly out of proportion to the event. Today's litigious climate has the pernicious effect of suppressing candor rather than bringing errors to the light of day.

Conclusion

The complexity of decision-making in healthcare management continues to increase, with more and more interested constituencies wanting to be part of the deliberations and subsequent actions taken. Regardless of the consensus of opinion on what should be done, in the final analysis *management* is accountable for decisions made: management must never allow itself to become a passive discipline.

This book is intended to serve as a "call to action" for healthcare managers throughout the world. Like many of society's institutions – religion, education, and government to name but a few – healthcare systems are suffering from a crisis of public confidence. While the overall challenges may seem insurmountable, healthcare managers have responsibility for their sphere of influence and can make changes that have a "ripple effect" on the system as a whole. We invite healthcare managers to serve as change agents. We challenge healthcare managers to adopt a personal action plan that includes six critical steps:

(1) View management mistakes differently – as *opportunities for improving* health-care, rather than failures

(2) Seriously consider the implementation of the *recommendations* offered throughout this book and highlighted in this closing chapter

(3) Take a *leadership role*, including admitting and disclosing one's own mistakes

(4) Establish policies and processes that make it clear to staff, physicians, govern-ance, and the public that you have a *learning organization* and then follow up to see that you do

(5) Cultivate a culture where *accountability is the norm*

(6) Be a *moral change agent* – one that models and encourages ethical conduct for the profession and for society.

The Association of Academic Health Centers (1990), in one of its policy statements, reminds us that: "the essence of a profession is that its members commit themselves to a set of standards higher than the morals of the market-place." There is both an irrefutable opportunity and an urgent imperative here for us to do this by morally managing the mistakes we make and using them to benefit the patients and communities we serve.

REFERENCES

Association of Academic Health Centers, 1990. "Conflicts of interest in academic health centers–policy paper: a report by the AHC Task Force on Science Policy." Washington, DC: ACHA: 6–7

Berger, P. and T. Luckmann, 1967. *The Social Construction of Reality*. Garden City, NY: Anchor Books

Blustein, J., L. Post, and N. Dubler, 2002. *Ethics for Health Care Organization: Theory, Case Studies, and Tools*. New York: United Hospital Fund of New York: **41**

Hofmann, P., 2003. "Management mistakes in healthcare: a disturbing silence,"*Cambridge Quarterly of Healthcare Ethics* **12(2)**: 201–202

Ignagni, K., 2003. "Moving beyond the blame game: reforming the malpractice system," *Frontiers of Healthcare Management* **20(1)**: 41

Institute of Medicine, 1999. To Err is Human. Building a Safer Health System (IOM report). Washington, DC: The Institute of Medicine and National Academy Press

Perry, F., 2001. The *Tracks We Leave: Ethics in Health Care Management*. Chicago: Health Administration Press

Taylor, M., 2003. "A question of integrity," *Modern Healthcare* **33(2)**: 6–7, 16

Worthley, J. A., 1997. *The Ethics of the Ordinary in Healthcare: Concepts and cases*. Chicago: Health Administration Press

Suggested further reading

Boyle, P., E. DuBose, S. Ellingson, D. Guinn, and D. McCurdy. *Organizational Ethics in Health Care: Principles, Cases, and Practical Solutions*. San Francisco: Jossey-Bass, 2001

Darr, K. *Ethics in Health Services Management*, 3rd edn. Baltimore, IMD: Health Professions Press, 1997.

Devettere, R. *Practical Decision Making in Health Care Ethics: Cases and Concepts*. Washington, DC: Georgetown University Press, 1995

Dracopoulou, S. (ed.). *Ethics and Values in Health care Management*. London: Routledge, 1998.

Dye, C. *Leadership in Health care: Values at the Top*. Chicago: Health Administration Press, 2000

Hall, R. *An Introduction to Healthcare Organizational Ethics*. Oxford: Oxford University Press, 2000

Hofmann, P. B. and W. A. Nelson. *Managing Ethically: An Executive's Guide*. Chicago: Health Administration Press, 2001.

Kleinke, J. *Bleeding Edge: The Business of Health Care in the New Century*. Gaithersburg, MD: Aspen Publishers, 1998

Institute of Medicine. *To Err is Human: Building a Safer Health System*. Washington, DC: Institute of Medicine and National Academy Press, 1999
Crossing the Quality Chasm. Washington, DC: National Academy Press, 2002

Kuczewski, M. and R. Pinkus. *An Ethics Casebook for Hospitals: Practical Approaches to Everyday Cases*. Washington, DC: Georgetown University Press, 1999

Leoyd, D., D. Wegmiller, and W. Wright. *Trials to Triumphs: Perspectives from Successful Healthcare Leaders*. Chicago: Health Administration Press, 2001

Loughlin, M. *Ethics and Mythology*. Abingdon, DC: Radcliffe Medical Press, 2001

Perry, F. *The Tracks We Leave: Ethics in Healthcare Management*. Chicago: Health Administration Press, 2001

Rakich, J., B. Longest, and K. Darr (eds). *Cases in Health Services Management*, 3rd edn. Baltimore, MD: Health Professions Press, 1995

Ross, A. *Cornerstones of Leadership for Healthcare Executives*. Ann Arbor, MI: Health Administration Press, 1992

Rubin, S. and L. Zoloth. *Margin of Error: The Ethics of Mistakes in the Practice of Medicine*. Hagerstown, MD: University Publishing Group, 2000

Spencer, E., A. Mills, M. Rorty, and P. Werhane. *Organization Ethics in Health Care*. Oxford: Oxford University Press, 2000

Stevens, R. *In Sickness and In Wealth: American Hospitals in the Twentieth Century*. New York: Basic Books, 1989

Worthley, J. A. *The Ethics of the Ordinary in Healthcare: Concepts and Cases*. Chicago: Health Administration Press, 1997

Index

Note: page numbers in *italics* refer to figures